C   .

JILL ECKERSLEY is a freelance .
experience of writing on health topics. She is a regular
contributor to women's and general-interest magazines,
including *Good Health*, *Bella*, *Ms London*, *Goodtimes*,
Woman's Realm and other titles. *Coping with Snoring and
Sleep Apnoea* (2003) was Jill's first book for Sheldon
Press. She lives beside the Regent's Canal in north London
with two cats.

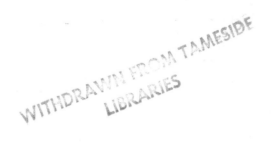

Overcoming Common Problems Series

For a full list of titles please contact
Sheldon Press, Marylebone Road, London NW1 4DU

The Assertiveness Workbook
A plan for busy women
JOANNA GUTMANN

Birth Over Thirty Five
SHEILA KITZINGER

Body Language
How to read others' thoughts by their
gestures
ALLAN PEASE

Body Language in Relationships
DAVID COHEN

Cancer – A Family Affair
NEVILLE SHONE

Coping Successfully with Hayfever
DR ROBERT YOUNGSON

Coping Successfully with Migraine
SUE DYSON

Coping Successfully with Pain
NEVILLE SHONE

**Coping Successfully with Your Irritable
Bowel**
ROSEMARY NICOL

Coping with Anxiety and Depression
SHIRLEY TRICKETT

Coping with Breast Cancer
DR EADIE HEYDERMAN

Coping with Bronchitis and Emphysema
DR TOM SMITH

Coping with Chronic Fatigue
TRUDIE CHALDER

Coping with Depression and Elation
DR PATRICK McKEON

Curing Arthritis Diet Book
MARGARET HILLS

Curing Arthritis – The Drug-Free Way
MARGARET HILLS

Depression
DR PAUL HAUCK

Divorce and Separation
Every woman's guide to a new life
ANGELA WILLANS

**Everything Parents Should Know About
Drugs**
SARAH LAWSON

Good Stress Guide, The
MARY HARTLEY

Heart Attacks – Prevent and Survive
DR TOM SMITH

Helping Children Cope with Grief
ROSEMARY WELLS

How to Improve Your Confidence
DR KENNETH HAMBLY

How to Interview and Be Interviewed
MICHELE BROWN AND GYLES
BRANDRETH

How to Keep Your Cholesterol in Check
DR ROBERT POVEY

How to Pass Your Driving Test
DONALD RIDLAND

**How to Start a Conversation and Make
Friends**
DON GABOR

How to Write a Successful CV
JOANNA GUTMANN

Hysterectomy
SUZIE HAYMAN

The Irritable Bowel Diet Book
ROSEMARY NICOL

Overcoming Guilt
DR WINDY DRYDEN

The Parkinson's Disease Handbook
DR RICHARD GODWIN-AUSTEN

Talking About Anorexia
How to cope with life without starving
MAROUSHKA MONRO

Think Your Way to Happiness
DR WINDY DRYDEN AND JACK
GORDON

Overcoming Common Problems

Coping with Childhood Asthma

Jill Eckersley

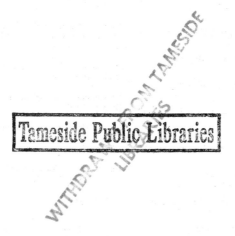

sheldon **PRESS**

First published in Great Britain in 2003 by
Sheldon Press
1 Marylebone Road
London NW1 4DU

British Library Cataloguing-in-Publication Data
A catalogue record for this book is available from the British Library

ISBN 0–85969–907–2

1 3 5 7 9 10 8 6 4 2

Typeset by Deltatype Ltd, Birkenhead, Wirral
Printed in Great Britain by Biddles Ltd, Guildford and King's Lynn
www.biddles.co.uk

Contents

	Acknowledgements	vi
	Introduction	vii
1	Asthma – A Modern Epidemic	1
2	The Heredity Factor	11
3	Asthma Triggers	17
4	Getting Professional Help	27
5	Managing Asthma	35
6	What Carers, Childminders and Teachers Should Know	47
7	'Will He Grow Out of It?'	56
8	Complementary Medicine	63
9	What about the Future?	73
10	Further Help	78
	Appendix 1: Vital Facts to Remember about Asthma	83
	Appendix 2: The Asthma Charter	85
	Index	87

Acknowledgements

I should like to thank the many health professionals, teachers, parents and young people with asthma who have generously helped me with this book. The British Lung Foundation and the British Thoracic Society were extremely supportive and without the expertise of the National Asthma Campaign the book would never have been written. Thanks, also, to Dr Andrew Bush and nurse Liz Biggart at the Royal Brompton Hospital, nurses Maureen Jenkins, Sue Clarke and Alison Summerfield, Dr Warren Lenny of the University Hospital of North Staffordshire and Dr Seif Shaheen of King's College, London. Many complementary therapists were equally generous with their time, as were the mums I spoke to who have learned to manage asthma on a day-to-day basis. They are the true experts.

Introduction

Perhaps you have picked up this book because you are a parent whose child has just been diagnosed asthmatic, and you are wondering exactly what that means. Or you are a teacher, nursery nurse or carer with an asthmatic child or children among your charges and you want to know more about the condition.

In that case, read on. This book aims to answer the most frequently asked questions about the condition, including what asthma is and how the treatments your child will be offered actually work. There is, as yet, no cure for asthma, but that doesn't mean it can't be managed. One of the experienced asthma nurses we interviewed said that the goal of modern asthma treatment is to enable affected children and their families to lead a normal life, with only minor adjustments to their lifestyle.

A National Asthma Campaign Scotland survey and report in 2002 identified five key concerns for parents:

- getting an accurate and early diagnosis;
- a lack of support from the child's school;
- negative experiences at Accident and Emergency (A&E) departments;
- substandard care from their GP;
- anxiety about medication.

All those concerns are currently being addressed by asthma experts, including those we spoke to for this book. Early diagnosis of asthma is difficult, especially in very young children, because there are so many other conditions like bronchiolitis and croup which can make children wheeze – one of the most characteristic symptoms of asthma. More and more schools now have policies in place to cater for children with asthma so that they can continue to benefit from their education with their asthma taken into account. Hospital A&E departments have also recognized that separate facilities for sick children, staffed by trained paediatric nurses, are the way forward. Many GP surgeries now offer specialist asthma clinics staffed by nurses with expertise in childhood asthma, including the latest and most up-to-date information about asthma medication and its possible side-effects. No one would claim that asthma care is perfect but it is improving all the time. Many doctors recognize that parents are often the best judges of their child's condition and stress that asthma management is about teamwork.

First of all, it might help to know you are far from being alone. In the UK, 1.4 million children are being treated for asthma, according to the National Asthma Campaign. It is almost three times more prevalent than any other childhood medical condition. There are 2.5 million parents of children with asthma in the UK.

Asthma impacts not only on the child, with frequent episodes of wheezy illness which can be frightening, time off school, visits to the GP and inhospitable A&E departments, but also on the family, leading to constant anxiety and sleepless nights. The National Asthma Campaign reports that a quarter of parents are woken one or more nights a week because of their child's asthma and one in six parents has had to take time off work to care for their asthmatic child. Schools, nurseries and playgroups are also affected, with many staff willing to help, but concerned that they have not received training and support from their employer, so that they are reluctant to administer medication or simply don't know what to do.

Both the National Asthma Campaign and the British Lung Foundation are carrying out research into the causes of asthma, campaigning for better resources and treatment, and offering support to affected families.

So what, exactly, is asthma, and why are so many of today's children affected by it? Read on ...

1

Asthma – A Modern Epidemic

Asthma is Britain's most common long-term childhood illness, according to the National Asthma Campaign. At present, the NAC estimate that one in five British children is diagnosed with asthma at some point in their life and that one British child in eight is currently being treated for asthma symptoms – coughing, wheezing and breathlessness. What's more, the numbers of children diagnosed with this condition seem still to be rising. In 1990, around 12 per cent of British under-5s were diagnosed with asthma. By 1998 the figure had risen to 21 per cent. Better diagnosis undoubtedly plays a part – there is some evidence that asthma was under-diagnosed in the past – but doesn't explain the huge rise in numbers.

It's not that asthma was unknown in the past. It is mentioned in ancient Chinese medical texts and was known to the ancient Greeks. The composers Vivaldi and Beethoven were asthmatics and so were Charles Dickens, Edward Lear and Benjamin Disraeli. Bob Hope, Elizabeth Taylor and Liza Minnelli also have asthma, as does DJ and TV presenter Chris Tarrant.

Asthma is a particular kind of chronic allergic reaction affecting the airways, leading to inflammation, narrowed airways and characteristic symptoms which include:

- wheezing;
- shortness of breath;
- tightness in the chest;
- coughing.

These symptoms are usually variable, intermittent, often worse at night, and can be provoked by various triggers including cigarette smoke, house-dust mites, contact with animals, and exercise.

All allergic reactions, including food allergy, eczema, hay-fever and the life-threatening anaphylaxis, are on the increase. In children aged between 5 and 14, asthma and other respiratory conditions now cause about one-fifth of all hospital in-patient admissions.

An international study in 1998 found that, in children aged 13–14, the UK had the highest incidence of 'severe wheeze' at 14.1 per cent. Australia, New Zealand and Canada also had a high incidence of wheeze, while countries like Finland, Belgium and Sweden had a low incidence at around 5 per cent. It is thought that the number of sufferers may have increased by as much as 50 per cent in more well-off countries over the last 25 years. Exactly why this should be so is not yet known. What is known is that some less developed parts of the world seem to have a low incidence of asthma. It is quite rare in rural Africa, China, Indonesia and among Australian aborigines and Inuit people. Various reasons for this have been suggested, from differences in climate to air pollution. However, the link is not a direct one. Research is going on all around the world to try and explain why some countries have high rates of asthma. Humid and subtropical Hong Kong seems to breed the same kind of house-dust mite as cool, temperate London, but Hong Kong youngsters have lower rates of asthma. Children in Sweden are more affected than those growing up in polluted Polish cities. After the fall of the Berlin Wall, East German levels of asthma and other allergic reactions took five years to catch up with West Germany and Britain. Something in our affluent Western lifestyle seems to be contributing to this rise but no one, as yet, has found out exactly what it is.

The British Lung Foundation says that much more research is needed into the factors which have caused the huge rise in the number of asthma cases, because no one single mechanism seems to fit all the available facts. Among the many different factors which are, or have been, implicated are:

- outdoor air pollution;
- indoor air pollution;
- smoking during pregnancy and children being exposed to smoke in the home;
- changes in diet;
- the Idling Immune System Theory;
- the 'Hygiene Hypothesis'.

Outdoor air pollution

Not everyone is equally sensitive to the different pollutants in the air we breathe, but there's some evidence that children are especially affected. Forty or fifty years ago, coal fires were responsible for most of the air pollution in Britain's cities. Polluted fog or 'smog' killed over 4,000 people in one notorious episode in London in 1952. Advances in smokeless fuels and Clean Air legislation removed those particular pollutants from the atmosphere, only for them to be replaced by traffic fumes which contain sulphur dioxide, nitrogen dioxide, carbon monoxide and ozone. According to the British Thoracic Society, these 'modern' pollutants are more likely to contribute to the rise in the number of asthma cases.

Sulphur dioxide is produced by power stations and diesel engines, and although levels of this chemical have fallen it's still a problem, as inhaling it can constrict the airways and make breathing difficult. Nitrogen dioxide, which is also produced by power stations and cars, irritates the lining of the bronchial tubes in the lungs. Ozone is formed when two kinds of traffic pollutants, oxides of nitrogen and hydrocarbons, are combined in sunlight. Ozone irritates the lungs and stings eyes, nose and throat. Carbon monoxide is an odourless, poisonous gas which comes from traffic fumes and cigarette smoke. None of these pollutants causes asthma on its own, but may act as a trigger in susceptible people and especially children. Babies in buggies and small children walking to school along busy, traffic-choked roads are probably breathing in a cocktail of polluted air from car exhausts which must make them vulnerable to respiratory problems, including asthma. According to environmental pressure group Friends of the Earth, traffic pollution is overwhelmingly the problem, especially in cities.

'Although modern cars are cleaner than they used to be, with advances like catalytic converters and lead-free petrol, there are far more cars on the roads and they are driving further, causing even more pollution,' says their spokesman.

Nor is it always possible to escape from traffic pollution by moving to the country. Because of the weather, pollution levels are sometimes higher in the countryside, when the prevailing winds blow the pollution from the cities. Teenage asthma seems to be higher in the country than in towns and there are more cases per head of population on the Isle of Skye than on the mainland! Apparently rural Oxfordshire and Somerset have both recorded extremely high ozone levels and the highest levels of all were recorded at an isolated nature reserve on the Sussex coast. These were probably caused by pollutants drifting over from Belgian or French cities.

Indoor air pollution

Most of the air we breathe contains very low levels of pollutants like dust, gases, mould and chemicals. In small amounts, these are harmless. However, trapped in a confined space like a well-insulated, centrally heated modern home, indoor pollution can sometimes cause breathing problems in susceptible people.

The best way to control indoor air pollution is to avoid or remove whatever is causing it, as well as making sure that rooms are properly ventilated. The most common indoor pollutants include tobacco smoke, animal dander (a mixture of hair and saliva which causes an allergic reaction), house-dust mites which are present in even the cleanest homes, mould and mildew which flourish in damp conditions, gases released by poorly maintained household appliances, and even the toxic chemicals found in some household cleaning products. One expert suggested that a possible cause for the increase in childhood asthma could be that today's children spend so much more time indoors. A combination of more home entertainment, with multiple TV channels, computers and games consoles, and parents' safety fears could be confining more youngsters to their houses. A study for the Children's Society in 1999 found that 80 per cent of parents think their children spend less time playing outside than they themselves did. Fewer children now walk to school than in 1990.

Smoking during pregnancy and children's exposure to smoke in the home

Sadly, and in spite of all the government health warnings, there is some evidence that young women of child-bearing age are actually smoking more – or at least, not giving up as much as men. About a third of pregnant women still smoke during their pregnancy. Only about a quarter of pregnant female smokers give up when they become pregnant, and most take up smoking again after they have had their babies. It is known that babies whose mothers smoked during pregnancy have an increased risk of developing asthma. Premature and low-birthweight babies are especially at risk. One study suggested that as many as one-third developed asthma during their first year. As more is learned about how the lungs of unborn babies develop, researchers have found that smokers' babies tend to have narrower airways which become blocked more easily.

'One of the few things that parents can do which we *know* reduces the risk of babies and children developing asthma is to give up smoking,' comments Dr Andrew Bush, Consultant Paediatrician at London's Brompton Hospital.

Childhood asthma is not always caused by inflammation. It is sometimes caused by things that happened before the child was born: for example, having a mum who smokes during pregnancy. My message to those planning a pregnancy would be: give up smoking. Even if your pregnancy is unplanned, and you don't find out you are pregnant for weeks, it's still worth giving up. The damage to the baby's developing airways seems to be done in the second half of pregnancy.

A new and very big research study in Australia found some evidence that babies whose mothers suffer from high blood pressure during pregnancy are more likely to develop asthma, although as yet no one seems to have worked out why this could be. Giving up smoking is the one thing we *know* could improve the respiratory health of babies and children.

Children whose parents are smokers are also at risk. Even though less than one-third of British adults now smoke, almost a half of the country's children live in a home where someone smokes. It has been worked out that a child whose parents smoke inhales the equivalent of 60–150 cigarettes'-worth of nicotine a year. A study of 4,000 under-5s found that children whose mothers smoked ten or more cigarettes a day had a higher rate of asthma and required more medication than the children of non-smokers. Children who are hospitalized because of their asthma and go home to a smoking household recover less well. The children's TV programme *Blue Peter* found in 1995 that three-quarters of asthmatic children said their symptoms were made worse in smoky atmospheres. One asthma nurse I spoke to said that, ideally, parents should give up smoking two years before they plan to try for a baby.

Although the relationship between tobacco smoke and asthma is a complex one, worldwide research over the last twenty years has produced evidence that passive smoking increases the risk of a child developing asthma and also makes the symptoms worse. Tobacco smoke contains tar, poisonous gases and toxic chemicals which can damage young lungs. Children whose parents and carers smoke are more at risk of cot death, meningitis and other chest infections as well as asthma.

Changes in diet

Those of us who keep up with the latest ideas on healthy eating know that eating our five portions of fruit and veg a day provides enough antioxidants to help prevent cancer and other degenerative diseases. It seems as though a diet rich in antioxidant vitamins and minerals could prevent asthma too. It is already known that adult asthmatics eat less of the antioxidant mineral selenium, although less is known about selenium intake in children. Interestingly, the amount of selenium eaten in Britain *has* dropped in the past ten years or so. That was when we stopped buying American wheat, which is grown in selenium-rich soil, and started buying the wheat for our bread from Europe. Researchers are still trying to establish whether there could be a link between low selenium intake and asthma.

Some complementary therapists say that excluding dairy products from the diet can help to reduce the number of asthma attacks. However, mainstream medicine is dubious about this, not least because it's vitally important for young children – many of whom may be faddy eaters anyway – to eat a healthy, balanced diet. The calcium in dairy products is vital for bone health and future growth.

'Allergen exclusion diets treble your shopping time because you have to read the small print on all the food labels,' comments Dr Andrew Bush.

If parents are especially concerned about the effect of diet on their child's asthma, they really should see a paediatric dietician rather than cutting a very important group of foods out of the child's diet. There is evidence that the calcium contained in milk and cheese is more effective at promoting bone health than calcium supplements.

Fish oils and apples have also been suggested as having a protective effect against asthma, and researchers are still trying to confirm this. Meanwhile the best advice seems to be to eat a sensible, balanced diet and not forget the five-a-day rule.

The Idling Immune System Theory

Something called the Idling Immune System Theory has also been suggested as a possible reason for the increase in asthma cases. The theory is that as today's children now suffer from fewer infectious diseases during childhood, their immune systems now target other organs, e.g. the lungs.

'It seems to be true that children with lots of siblings who pass on colds and other infections, and children who spend time with other children in day-care, are less likely to develop asthma,' says Dr Bush.

The way this is said to work is that the white cells in the immune system can either develop as TH-1 types, which fight infection, or TH-2 types which seem to cause allergy problems. The reason for this is evolutionary. Humans used to suffer from lots of parasites which TH-2 cells were good at fighting. Cells which at one time would have been fighting infections are now becoming TH-2 types, leading to more asthma and other allergic conditions.

It has to be said, though, that this is still a contentious theory. It is based on work with laboratory mice, and is probably also true for humans, but it's something that even the experts are still arguing about.

It could, however, help to explain why asthma is relatively rare in Third World countries, where people's immune systems are still kept busy dealing with life-threatening infectious diseases.

The 'Hygiene Hypothesis'

The 'Hygiene Hypothesis' states that we now live in such clean homes that we are vulnerable to all kinds of allergies that wouldn't have been a problem in the past. Work is even being done on an anti-asthma vaccine based on dirt! This might explain why children brought up on farms tend to be asthma-free – not just because they are exposed to allergens like animal dander but because farmyards are much less sterile than other environments. Again, this is just a theory.

Where asthma is concerned, there are still a lot of areas of uncertainty. It is still not known for sure whether exposing children to more allergens – pet hair, for example – makes them more or less likely to develop conditions like asthma. According to the British Thoracic Society, there are a number of scientific studies suggesting that close contact with a cat or dog during very early infancy reduces the chances of the child developing asthma or allergy later.

No child can live in a totally sterile environment, and even if it were possible it might not help. It seems to depend on what actually triggers asthma attacks in individuals. While 25 per cent of the *Blue Peter* children said that contact with pets made their asthma worse (and some very susceptible children develop 'schoolday asthma' simply by sitting next to classmates who have pets at home, especially cats), that still leaves 75 per cent who said it didn't. Asthma is very much an individual problem.

'We are still trying to understand the reasons for the rise in the number of cases,' admits Dr Seif Shaheen, an epidemiologist from King's College in London.

Once we can identify the causes we might be able to prevent asthma, but at the moment we just don't have all the answers we need. The idea that children are developing asthma because they are no longer in contact with so many infectious diseases sounds plausible – except that the numbers of cases of infectious diseases began to drop in the 1950s, not in the last ten years. There are also many studies suggesting that contact with animals has a protective effect, rather than causing asthma, suggesting that heavy exposure to animal hair might actually make the immune system more tolerant. Over-use of antibiotics has also been blamed, as has vaccination, but there is no really convincing evidence for this, in spite of the anti-vaccine lobby.

A report from east Germany in April 2003 suggested that there may be a link between childhood asthma and use of the Pill. In a group of 2,754 children who were studied, 5.6 per cent of those whose mothers used the Pill before they became pregnant, and 7.1 per cent of those whose mothers used the Pill after the birth, had asthma, compared with 4.4 per cent of those whose mothers were not Pill users. However, even the doctors who conducted the study admitted that other, external factors could be involved, and other studies have found no link between the Pill and asthma.

'There are many clues suggesting that factors before birth may influence the development of childhood asthma,' says Dr Shaheen. 'Other studies have looked at pregnancy complications, infections from which pregnant women have suffered, even Caesarean deliveries, but the true cause is still a mystery.'

Research by the British Lung Foundation has confirmed that asthma is not one single disease, but a combination of breathing disorders with similar symptoms. Knowing this means that treatment can be tailored to a child's individual problems, but different descriptions and diagnoses can cause confusion for parents and carers. You may be told that your child has 'wheeze' or 'wheezy bronchitis' rather than asthma.

It can be extremely frightening to witness your child having an asthma attack, particularly the first time it happens.

'Josh had breathing problems from when he was about five months old,' says his mother Denise.

We have asthma, eczema and hay-fever in the family and his older brother and sister are also affected. Even as a baby Josh had eczema on his chest and torso and he wheezed really badly. My doctor diagnosed bronchiolitis at first, and he was 'chesty' as a baby and toddler. When I took him to the clinic for his 3-year-old check-up he became very, very breathless and his nose began to bleed. Another complication was that when he had an attack he was always sick. It was as though his body could only deal with one problem at once – his breathing difficulties – and his digestive system just couldn't cope. He had to be rushed to hospital, put on a drip, and treated with steroids. I was told that his oxygen levels were way, way down from the 100 per cent they should have been if his lungs had been working properly. He was in hospital for four or five days while they tried to get the steroid dose right to control his asthma.

When he was very small the steroids seemed to work well, but as he got older they just seemed to stop working. By the time he was 8 or so he had had so much time off school that I was worried about his education as well as his health. My GP gave him a different inhaler and that worked for a time. Then we were referred to a hospital clinic and eventually to the paediatric asthma clinic at the Royal Brompton Hospital in London. There, the doctors established that he was one of the rare children who did not respond well to steroids, either inhaled or in tablet form, so now he has a 24-hour pump which contains terbutaline, a well-known bronchodilator. Before he had the pump he could hardly walk without getting breathless but now he is able to exercise again providing he doesn't overdo it.

When you first hear the word 'asthma' you may know nothing more than the basic fact that asthmatic children have trouble breathing and that they have to use an inhaler. So what, exactly, is asthma?

A working definition might be that asthma is a condition in which breathing becomes difficult because of a narrowing of the airways which varies over short periods of time. The airways become inflamed, irritated, twitchy and sore. They also produce more mucus, which obstructs breathing and causes the familiar symptoms of coughing, wheezing and breathlessness.

However, there are respiratory conditions other than asthma which can cause coughing and wheezing, for example 'viral-associated wheeze' which, as its name suggests, is caused by a virus. Another possibility is bronchiolitis, another viral disorder which is very common in small children. The flu-like virus attacks the bronchioles which are narrow airways within the lungs and makes them ultra-sensitive and full of mucus. Some children need to be hospitalized. Croup is another possibility. It is caused by a virus which affects the back of the throat and the windpipe, causing breathlessness, hoarseness and a characteristic 'barking' cough.

Breathlessness in young children, especially after exercise, should always be investigated whether the child is wheezing and coughing or not.

Because there are several different conditions that can cause children to wheeze, it is unlikely that a baby or small child will be diagnosed with classic allergic asthma before she is about 3. That doesn't mean that small children don't have distressing episodes of wheezing and breathlessness before that age, just that doctors can't be certain of the diagnosis.

'Asthma is not something which doctors can do a blood test for, and diagnosis in young children is especially difficult,' says Professor Martin Partridge, Chief Medical Adviser to the National Asthma Campaign.

Wheezing in young children may be caused by a virus or they may have especially small airways, so it is often not possible to say with certainty that a small child has classic allergic asthma. Nor can doctors tell at that stage whether he will or won't grow out of it.

As yet, there is no 'cure' for asthma. It's a condition that children and their families have to live with. However, with correct diagnosis, careful management, the right treatment, and a few adjustments to family lifestyle, children with asthma should be able to live a normal life.

2

The Heredity Factor

Asthma is caused by a combination of inherited and environmental factors. In other words, your asthmatic child will probably have inherited a **tendency** to asthma, and environmental factors like a smoky atmosphere will act as **triggers** (see Chapter 3) which cause asthma to develop, or lead to asthma attacks. The tendency for a particular individual to develop asthma or other allergic conditions is called **atopy**. According to the British Thoracic Society, a family history of atopy is the most important, clearly defined risk factor for atopy in children. However, it is not unknown for asthma suddenly to appear in a family where there is no history of it, or of any other allergic illness.

A 'complex inheritable condition'

Doctors and scientists have been studying the causes of asthma for ninety years and still haven't come to any firm conclusions – except to say that asthma and other allergic conditions run in families! However, it is known as a 'complex inheritable condition' – like diabetes and high blood pressure – which means that a number of genes, and not just one, contribute to an individual's susceptibility to asthma. In order to find out more about exactly how asthma is inherited, doctors in the 1970s studied pairs of identical twins and found that allergic conditions were more common in identical than fraternal twins. However, they also found that not all twins developed the same allergies, although if one had an allergic condition, the other was quite likely to have one too.

Our genes are located on chromosomes, with each chromosome containing hundreds of genes. More recent research has implicated several possible chromosomes as locations for asthma genes, and research is ongoing.

In 2002, scientists at the University of Southampton succeeded in identifying at least one gene which seems to play a key role in the development of asthma. This gene is called ADAM33 and is found on chromosome 20. It relates to the development of over-responsive airways (the inflammation which characterizes asthma). According to researchers this discovery could lead to new diagnoses and treatments in the future. However, we still do not have a complete picture of exactly how asthma is inherited.

Asthma is an allergic response, and most childhood asthma is caused by an allergy. Doctors treating children with respiratory problems like coughing, wheezing and breathlessness will ask parents if there is any history of asthma or other allergic disease in the family. That doesn't just mean asthma, it also includes eczema, hay-fever, food allergies or rhinitis (a permanently itchy, streaming nose). All these conditions are different manifestations of the same problem with the body's immune system.

If either or both parents have asthma or a related condition, the chances of children developing asthma are higher. According to the McGovern Asthma and Allergy Clinic in the USA, if both parents have asthma or another allergic condition, the chances of their children also having it are as high as 75 per cent. If only one parent has an allergic condition, the chances go down to around 40 per cent. On the other hand, 38 per cent of people with allergy problems, including asthma, have no family history. If only the mother has asthma, the chances of the child developing it are higher than if only the father has it.

Can asthma be prevented?

Parents often want to know if there is anything they can do to prevent their children inheriting their asthma. Although the precise causes of asthma are not known in every case, there do seem to be precautions parents-to-be can take when they know there is asthma in the family. For example:

- While you are pregnant, minimize your exposure to allergens like pollen and house-dust mite. If you are an asthma or hay-fever sufferer, you will probably be doing this anyway.
- Don't keep furry or feathery pets. Again, people suffering from allergies are unlikely to do this.
- There is little evidence that changing your diet during pregnancy will prevent your baby from developing asthma. A healthy well-balanced diet is best for you and your baby. Contact the WellBeing/Sainsbury's Eating for Pregnancy Helpline (address on p. 80) for the latest information on healthy eating during pregnancy.
- It's worth noting that there is some evidence that peanut allergy may develop in the womb. If you have a family history of asthma,

eczema, allergy or hay-fever, it is recommended that you don't eat peanuts or peanut products during pregnancy or while you are breast-feeding.

- Try to breast-feed your baby for at least four months. Some, but not all, studies have shown that breast-feeding in the first few months may reduce a child's chances of developing allergies, including asthma. It's unlikely that your baby will be allergic to your own breast milk, although some babies are allergic to one or other of the proteins in cow's milk. Some asthmatic mothers worry that their asthma medication could affect the baby, but normal doses of inhaled steroids – the most usual treatment for asthma – do not enter the bloodstream so they are not found in breast milk. If a breast-feeding mother has to take steroid tablets for asthma, the quantities found in breast milk are too small to have any harmful effect on the baby. If you are bottle-feeding your baby, take your doctor's or practice nurse's advice on the best formula to use.

- Try to minimize your baby's exposure to cough and cold germs until he is six months old at least. Researchers at Imperial College, London, have found that delaying infection with cold viruses beyond the first six months of life could make a real difference to the child's health. Cold viruses can lead to bronchiolitis, and around four out of ten babies who suffer from bronchiolitis are later affected by wheezy and asthmatic illness. It appears that the immune system deals with cold viruses differently at different stages of life.

- Give up smoking. Although there are differences of opinion about some of the causes of asthma, and conflicting research findings which make for confusion, asthma specialists agree that the one thing that would improve children's respiratory health would be for all those who come into contact with children to be non-smokers. It's tough, if you are a nicotine addict, but there's no getting away from it! A study by Professor Jean Golding of Bristol University looked at 14,000 mothers in the Bristol area in the early 1990s and asked them to keep a diary of their babies' health for six months after birth. Results showed that the longer the mother continued to smoke, the more likely it was that her baby would wheeze or become breathless in its first six months. Smoking from mid-pregnancy onwards was associated with wheezing attacks in the baby. Giving up smoking at *any* stage of pregnancy reduces the risk of the baby suffering from wheezing and breathlessness.

Understanding an asthma attack

In order to understand what's happening when your child has an asthma attack, you need to know a bit about the immune system and its responses.

'Allergy is a disease of the immune system,' explains Maureen Jenkins, who is an Allergy Nurse Consultant.

The immune system is there to fight viruses, bacteria and parasites which it perceives as harmful invaders. What we call an allergic response happens when the immune system over-reacts to ordinary, non-harmful substances.

In normal circumstances, your immune system will produce antibodies of various types to fight off infection. The type which causes an allergic reaction is called Immunoglobulin E or IgE. If these antibodies appear in the white cells in your airways they will become sore and inflamed, and will produce more mucus than usual, narrowing them and leading to breathing difficulties and wheezing – the classic symptoms of asthma. IgE antibodies in the nose will give you hay-fever, in the skin will give you a rash or eczema, or in the gut will give you a stomach upset.

All these allergic reactions are related, which explains why children with asthma are more likely to get other allergies as well – although they may not. It also explains why children can 'inherit' classic allergic asthma in families where no one else has it – although parents or other relations may suffer from other allergies, for instance hay-fever or eczema, instead.

Asthma and anaphylaxis

Allergic reactions vary from those which are mildly inconvenient – a runny nose or a skin rash which clears up as soon as you learn to avoid the allergen which is causing it – to the life-threatening, which is known as anaphylaxis. This an extremely severe allergic reaction which can, if untreated, prove fatal. The most common causes of anaphylaxis include foods like peanuts, other nuts, fish, shellfish, dairy products and eggs. Non-food causes include latex, wasp and bee stings and some pharmaceutical drugs such as penicillin. In some extremely sensitive people, even a minute trace of the substance can cause swelling of the mouth and throat, severe asthma, a speeded-up heart rate, a drop in blood pressure, choking and collapse. For anyone prone to anaphylaxis, adrenaline injection kits are available in two strengths, adult and junior.

Patricia has mild allergic asthma herself. Her teenage son David has asthma and is at risk of anaphylaxis and Patricia has learned over the years that the two conditions are often linked.

'American research suggests that most fatal cases of anaphylaxis are in children with pre-existing asthma,' she says.

Almost as soon as David was born I noticed that he had problems with his skin which looked like eczema. My GP suggested that I went on a dairy-free diet as I was breast-feeding. Once I did that the skin problems cleared up but David seemed to have a lot of breathing problems including a couple of 'asthmatic' episodes before he was a year old. He became very hyperactive, his breathing was rapid and he went blue around the mouth. He was rushed to hospital where a nebulizer was used to get the drugs into him.

He also proved to be severely allergic to milk and eggs. In what was called an 'egg challenge', raw egg was sprayed into his mouth and he promptly went into anaphylactic shock! He had frequent asthma attacks until he was given preventer medication in the form of a steroidal inhaler called beclomethasone which was very effective. I was concerned at first about the possible side-effects of the long-term use of steroids but they haven't caused David any problems.

We found that his asthma was much worse in winter and not too much bother in summer so we were able to adjust his medication accordingly. Now, his asthma seems well controlled. His other allergies, to eggs, wasp and bee stings, don't seem to affect him too badly now he is older, but he still has problems with cow's milk. He has been hospitalized twice in the last year. Once, he ate a Murray Mint. He spat it out almost immediately, saying it didn't taste right, but he still went into anaphylactic shock. I later rang the manufacturers who told me that the mints were produced on the same production line as Butter Mints and the products must have been mixed up. The other time he ate a bit of a Mr Kipling apple pie which we later discovered had a 0.006 per cent milk protein content. Even that was enough to cause a reaction.

David's story illustrates just how careful those with severe allergic reactions have to be. The Anaphylaxis Campaign (address on p. 79) was formed in early 1994 by a small group of concerned parents, among them David Reading, whose 17-year-old daughter Sarah tragically died in 1993 after eating a piece of lemon meringue pie in a department store restaurant. The pie contained traces of peanut, to which Sarah was allergic, and resulted in her suffering a fatal anaphylactic shock. The campaign aims to raise awareness of the problem and is fighting for better research and treatment. Thankfully it is only a minority of asthmatic children who suffer such severe reactions. Parents – and, as they grow older, children themselves – soon learn which factors set off an attack of coughing, wheezing or breathlessness. These factors, known as **triggers**, are different for each child and we shall be looking at them in the next chapter.

3

Asthma Triggers

Prevention is always better than cure. If your child is chesty and you suspect that she may be asthmatic, it makes sense to avoid the triggers that seem to lead to an episode of wheezing, coughing or breathlessness. The only way to find out just what these are is by observation. Sometimes it's obvious what is upsetting your child, but you can also be taken by surprise.

'At first, I thought Matthew's asthma was only going to be a problem when he had a cold,' says his mother Julie.

> It started when he was 2 and had a bad attack of wheezing and breathlessness. Luckily our GP takes a special interest in asthma and Matt's wheezing was soon well controlled using a nebulizer and then a Ventolin inhaler with spacer and mask when he was little.
>
> Exercise seemed to play a part, too, and he sometimes had to sit out of football when he was at school, but luckily his teachers were very understanding.
>
> We live in the countryside and Matt's dad is a gamekeeper. Although Matt was perfectly all right around cats and dogs, he once came into contact with a wild deer. His eyes swelled up and he began to wheeze so badly that he had to go to Accident and Emergency, where steroids and anti-histamines were prescribed for him. We have two horses, and Matt is OK with my Arab/Welsh cross but wheezes if he goes too near the Shetland pony, which has a thick, woolly coat. He had a bad reaction to a friend's guinea-pig, too. Asthma triggers seem to be different for everyone.

Allergy testing

Allergy testing is a possibility and can be arranged by your GP, but neither 'skin prick testing', in which a minute amount of the allergen is applied to the child's skin, nor blood tests are 100 per cent accurate. Health professionals recommend caution in dealing with independent clinics which claim to offer allergy testing, sometimes by post. Some are reputable but others are less so. With commercial companies you should always ask yourself what they have to gain.

The answer is often a lot of money from the pockets of worried and confused patients. All treatments should be backed up by proper scientific evidence, normally from clinical trials involving large numbers of patients with the results published in reputable medical journals. Sadly, with some so-called 'allergy clinics' it's more a case of 'buyer beware'. Some people are told that 'tests' show an allergic response to a huge variety of foods, which leads to them putting their child on a very restricted and unhealthy diet.

Asthma nurse Liz Biggart of London's Brompton Hospital says:

> Allergy testing can be helpful in a specialized setting, but it isn't the whole story. A test can show whether the body sets up an immune reaction to a particular substance and how severe the reaction is. It could mean that we can say that the family should think about re-homing the cat, and could confirm what parents have already observed about the triggers for a child's asthma attacks. In the end, identifying triggers comes down to personal experience. If a child's cough is worse at night, that could indicate that the main problem is dust mites in the bedding. Or, if a child's asthma is worse in summer, it might suggest that pollen is a problem so it would help to keep the windows closed when the pollen count is high. Most children have multiple triggers anyway. If you take away one or two of the worst ones and the child is on the right medication, the impact of the triggers will be reduced right down to an acceptable level.

Triggers are different for everyone and reactions to well-established triggers can be more or less serious in individual children. Some highly sensitive children will begin to wheeze if they come into contact with someone whose clothes have been contaminated with animal dander, for instance. Others can stroke or play with animals for some time before they start to show any ill-effects. You may find that your child is affected by multiple triggers, like Jane's son Luke, who was first admitted to hospital suffering from respiratory problems at the age of just six weeks. He is now 10.

'Everywhere he goes has to be vetted,' says Jane.

> We have found over the years that his asthma is brought on by contact with pets, but also by his chemical sensitivities. That means no perfumes in the house, or polishes, spray deodorants, paint, house-plants or flowers. House-dust mites are a problem for Luke as well. Our house has wooden floors instead of carpets,

blinds instead of curtains, and leather armchairs. I don't use any chemical cleaners and I decorate when he is away spending time with his dad. Even my sister has had her carpets specially treated for house-dust mite. I buy new pillows every year and take our own anti-allergy bedding everywhere we go. I damp-dust and do the hoovering when Luke is at school and make sure the house is thoroughly aired. Pollen is a trigger for him, too, so we have to sleep with the windows closed in summer as pollen descends at night. If it's very hot, we use a fan to circulate the air. We have had to make a lot of changes but they do seem to have worked.

Among the most common triggers for asthma attacks in children are colds and other respiratory infections, passive smoking, allergens like house-dust mite and pet dander, exercise and stress. Less common triggers include cold air, certain drugs and food allergies.

Let's consider these in turn.

Colds and respiratory infections

Most children's asthma gets worse when they have a cold, meaning that symptoms which should clear up within six or seven days can linger for weeks. This is because the cold virus irritates the already sensitive airways, producing mucus and inflammation. Anything that does this causes the airways to tighten and makes breathing more difficult. As we have already seen, infections like bronchiolitis can switch on an initial episode of asthma-type symptoms in susceptible children.

Obviously, it's very difficult to keep babies and small children away from cold viruses altogether, and there's plenty of evidence that this would not be desirable anyway. A study at London's Imperial College found that keeping young babies – up to six months old – free from colds improved their health in childhood, but the general consensus among chest physicians seems to be that children need to be exposed to common viruses in order to build up their immunity.

'Normal exposure seems to be better for children's health,' says asthma nurse Liz Biggart.

You can't stop your child developing asthma by keeping him in a sterile environment. Up to the age of about 5, children's immune systems are still developing. Atopic children may benefit from

19

being exposed to cold viruses in the family and at school, because it helps their body to build up antibodies.

There's some evidence that breast-feeding for at least four months helps to protect babies.

Although you can't protect your children from minor childhood ailments completely, you can, of course, do your best to make sure they eat a healthy diet, rich in immune-boosting vitamins like Vitamin C. Making your children eat their greens is sometimes easier said than done, as every parent knows. These days, though, so many different fruits and veggies are available in the shops that you are sure to find something your child enjoys. If she turns her nose up at vegetables, try turning them into a puree or home-made vegetable soup. Fruit can be puréed, too, or enjoyed in the form of juice. Children tend to be conservative eaters, liking what they know. If they have been offered peeled and cored apples, strawberries, seedless grapes, lightly steamed carrots or broccoli florets, instead of chocolate and biscuits, from babyhood, they are more likely to grow up with healthy eating habits.

Passive smoking

Passive smoking is a scientifically proven irritant, which is not surprising when you realize what a cocktail of toxic chemicals tobacco smoke contains. Smokers may already know that they are inhaling a lethal mixture including nicotine, which as well as being addictive increases the heart rate and blood pressure. Nicotine is also an insecticide. Cigarettes contain tar, which is a mixture of cancer-causing chemicals, and carbon monoxide, the poisonous gas found in car exhaust fumes and faulty gas heaters, which is a known killer.

However, smokers may not realize that among the other chemicals in tobacco smoke are benzene, a gas found in petrol fumes which is known to cause leukaemia; ethanol, used in anti-freeze; ammonia, which is used in anti-personnel sprays and cleaning products; formaldehyde, which is embalming fluid; hydrogen cyanide, an industrial pollutant; toluene, an industrial solvent; and the insecticide DDT. It isn't hard to see why these substances need to be kept well away from babies and children, whether or not they have been diagnosed asthmatic.

Children, whose airways are narrower than adults' because they are still growing, are particularly affected by smoky atmospheres, and asthmatic children whose airways are already sensitized and 'twitchy' suffer most of all. 'Side stream' smoke makes up 85 per cent of the smoke in a smoky environment. This is the smoke that comes from the end of a lit cigarette or cigar, in contrast to the smoke actually breathed in and out by the smoker, known as 'mainstream smoke'. Side stream smoke is said to contain a higher concentration of toxic chemicals. As we've already seen, children whose parents smoke inhale the equivalent of 60–150 cigarettes'-worth of nicotine a year.

Your asthmatic child might react to smoke in the atmosphere immediately, but if he doesn't it doesn't mean that it isn't harmful. The long-term effect of passive smoking is likely to make his asthma worse.

It's obviously best to keep your asthmatic child away from smoky places, and fortunately the risks of passive smoking are now so well documented that there are more and more non-smoking areas in shops, restaurants and transport. Some local health authorities produce lists of smoke-free zones in hotels and places of entertainment. You can check these out on the Action on Smoking and Health website, address on p. 80.

Having an asthmatic child might be just the spur you need to turn you and your partner into non-smokers, even if you have had trouble giving up before. You will, of course, be benefiting your own health as well as your child's. Ask your doctor or pharmacist for advice on giving up or call one of the helplines listed on p. 80. Thousands of people have managed to give up, and so can you. What better incentive could there be than making a difference to your child's health?

While you are still a smoker, try to maintain a smoke-free environment at home if you can. Keep any smoke well away from your child's bed or cot and from the areas where he eats or plays. The smoke from a single cigarette lingers in the air for two and a half hours, even if the windows are open. Maybe you could restrict your smoking to one room, which you will need to keep well ventilated, or even smoke outside.

When friends or family who are still smoking come to visit, explain that smoking brings on your child's asthma and ask them to have a cigarette before they arrive. Hopefully, grandparents and friends who care about your child will be willing to restrict their smoking in this way. They might even be inspired to give up too!

The same applies if you have to visit smokers' houses. If you say that keeping your child away from smoky atmospheres is on doctor's orders, they are less likely to feel that you are being unnecessarily fussy. Passive smoking makes children, especially asthmatic children, ill!

It goes without saying that you should try not to smoke at all in the car. The effects of passive smoking in such a confined space are even more harmful, and breathing cigarette fumes in addition to the smell of petrol can make children car-sick.

House-dust mites

According to a study at London's St Bartholomew's Hospital, about one-third of the population is sensitive to house-dust mites, although not all those actually develop allergy symptoms. Like other allergies, this seems to be an increasing problem.

House-dust mites are tiny creatures, too small to be seen with the naked eye, which live and multiply in the warm, humid conditions of our modern homes. They are particularly common in our beds and bedrooms, but also in carpets and on soft furnishings. They feed on tiny flakes of human skin and leave droppings which can cause allergic reactions ranging from rhinitis – a runny nose – to asthma attacks.

House-dust mites are present in their millions even in the cleanest of homes, and today's centrally heated, well-insulated, draught-free houses provide an ideal environment for them to thrive. Fortunately, if you suspect that house-dust mites are a trigger for your child's asthma attacks there is quite a lot you can do to minimize the amount of allergen in your home.

Many of the changes you might need to make are cheap and easy, so start with them. Reduce the amount of damp in your home by opening windows after activities like cooking, washing and bathing. Don't dry clothes in bedrooms and living-rooms. If you have to dry them in the kitchen, bathroom or utility room, keep a window open and the door to the rest of the house shut so that the damp doesn't spread. Allow beds to air in the morning before making them up.

Other changes are slightly more expensive. You could, for instance, consider replacing carpets and rugs with plain wooden floors, and curtains with window blinds, especially in bedrooms. You can buy special allergy-proof bedding which forms a dust mite-proof barrier from companies like The Healthy House (see p. 80). If you are thinking of buying new furniture, consider materials like leather, cane, wood and canvas, which don't harbour dust mites.

You can vacuum regularly with one of the vacuum cleaners with a HEPA (high-energy particulate air) filter. These cleaners are specially designed to filter out dust-mite particles and pollen. The National Asthma Campaign and Allergy UK (addresses on pp. 78 and 79) have information about these. Ordinary vacuuming simply moves the dust around, so don't do it while your asthmatic child is in the room, and keep the windows open. Always dust with a damp cloth. Have as few dust-collecting ornaments, pictures and cushions as you can. Bed-linen and children's soft toys should be washed regularly at a temperature of 60°. Toys can even be kept in the freezer to kill off any mites. Turn the central heating down as low as is comfortable, especially in bedrooms. Keep your home well ventilated by opening windows in the daytime, even in winter. Vacuum the mattress every time you change the bed. The average person loses 500–900 ml of perspiration every day and in a cosy bed in a warm room this is a perfect environment for house-dust mites.

You will probably have to wait a couple of months before you notice any difference in your child's symptoms after making these changes. Remember that she may be sensitive to more than one asthma trigger.

Animal dander

Having animals around the home can be a contentious issue for families with asthmatic children. Of course, if your child can't be in the presence of anything furry or feathered without developing severe asthma symptoms, the rule is simple: no pets. However, the idea that animals equals allergies can lead to a lot of heartbreak in families for whom Fluffy or Fido is one of the family. All animal welfare groups and rescue centres are familiar with the scenario where animals are given up for re-homing because of an allergy – either real or suspected.

If you already have asthma or allergies in the family, think carefully before getting a pet. It is not usually the fur or feathers which cause the problem, but 'dander', an allergen which comes from a combination of hair and saliva. Usually, cats evoke the most serious allergic response in sensitive children, followed by male rabbits, birds, dogs, horses, guinea-pigs, hamsters and other small mammals. Again, the response is an individual one. Children who can't tolerate cats might be able to cope with a dog, or perhaps a female rabbit. Even particular breeds may make a difference. Cats like the curly-coated Devon or Cornish Rex, or dogs such as poodles, may be less likely to bring on a child's asthma. Allergen production increases with the pet's age, so that children who can tolerate a puppy or kitten in the house may become allergic as the animal grows.

If you do keep your pet, you will need to pay scrupulous attention to home hygiene, following all the tips in the section on house-dust mites and keeping the animal out of your child's bedroom. A new generation of 'pet wipes' is now available which claim to reduce the amount of animal dander in the air to manageable levels. It is sometimes suggested that you bathe your pet regularly as well as washing its bedding and toys. Some dogs enjoy a bath but very few cats do – unless you have a Turkish Van cat as they are very keen swimmers! Bathing a cat once a week is said to reduce the amount of allergen in the home by as much as 90 per cent.

Cats Protection, the cat welfare charity (address on p. 79), also produces a free leaflet, *Do You Have Asthma?* They recommend grooming the cat outdoors, making sure it doesn't have fleas (scratching spreads the allergens around), wiping it over with a damp cloth occasionally and, above all, being certain that cat dander is the problem before putting your pet and your family through the stress of re-homing. It's worth remembering, too, that the presence of pets in the home does not cause asthma in non-susceptible people, so don't assume that just because you are pregnant the animal will have to go. As I've already noted, there is some evidence that children brought up in close contact with animals are *less* likely to develop asthma and other allergies.

Exercise

Exercise can bring on asthma attacks in some children. In the very young, one of the first symptoms parents may notice is that the child isn't running around and playing as much as before. He may tire easily, get breathless, and want to be carried. Breathlessness after ordinary exercise in young children should always be investigated by a health professional, whether or not it is accompanied by asthma-like symptoms of coughing and wheezing.

Exercise is vitally important for everyone, including, of course, growing children. It promotes normal, healthy growth and fitness and enables children to join in with their friends and have fun. This is just as important for children suffering from asthma as it is for any other children, and proper asthma management aims to ensure that children with asthma don't have to avoid exercise. Once your child has been prescribed her medication, in the form of 'preventer' and 'reliever' inhalers (see Chapter 5), make sure both you and she understand how to use them properly. If she takes her preventer as directed, every day, with a top-up puff or two of the reliever before she begins to play games or run around, she should be able to take part in normal exercise without wheezing. If she can't, perhaps her medication needs adjusting. Check with your GP or asthma nurse.

Swimming is a particularly good exercise for children with asthma. It's fun, it uses all the muscles, and the warm, damp atmosphere is unlikely to bring on an asthma attack.

Stress

Stress and excitement can be a common trigger, both in younger and older children. Toddler tantrums can sometimes result in an asthma attack, which can be distressing for both you and your child. Make sure you always have his medication handy. Stress can be good and bad – the excitement of a big event like a party or a family wedding or the worry of exams can also be an asthma trigger. If this seems to be the case for your child, make sure he is taking the medication as directed and also look at ways of coping psychologically. Relaxation techniques can be helpful.

Cold air

Some children seem to cough and wheeze if they go out into cold air. This is a natural, if exaggerated, response – people with healthy airways find their chests feel tight if they go out into the icy air of a Siberian winter. It's a protective mechanism. However, that doesn't mean children who react like this should stay indoors. A puff of their 'reliever' medication and a scarf over their face to warm up the air before it's breathed in should help.

Other triggers

Food allergies are a rare cause of asthma in young children. If your child seems to wheeze after he has eaten a particular food – dairy products and eggs are among the commoner ones – make a note of it when it happens and discuss it with your GP or asthma nurse.

The weather can make a difference, too. If your child's asthma is worse in spring and summer it could be pollen-related and your doctor may prescribe anti-histamines (hay-fever medication). Weather reports often give details of the pollen count and especially high ozone levels (see Chapter 1) for the benefit of asthma and allergy sufferers. Occasionally, medicines prescribed for other conditions may cause asthma symptoms, so if your child is prescribed anything always tell the doctor or pharmacist that she is asthmatic.

As girls reach puberty they may find that asthma attacks occur more often just before their periods. Asthma is more common in boys than girls, but at puberty more girls tend to develop asthma for the first time so that by the age of 18 asthma is more common in girls. It seems that hormones have some effect but what actually happens is not yet clearly understood.

If your daughter feels that her asthma is affected by her monthly cycle, it's a good idea for her to make a note in her diary of what's happening. If, after a few months, there seems to be a pattern, consult your GP or asthma nurse who may suggest she takes extra preventer treatment when her period is due. Stress (see above) may play a part here too. Young teenagers have a lot of changes to cope with all at once – new schools, exam choices, changing relation-ships. Sympathy, understanding and a listening ear, as well as exercise and relaxation, can help here.

Identifying the triggers for your child's asthma and avoiding them as far as possible will help you all to feel that you are controlling the condition, rather than letting it control you. Remember that the aim of asthma treatment is not so much a cure as an ability to lead a normal or near-normal life.

4

Getting Professional Help

If there is asthma in the family it's important that you have a good relationship with your family doctor. Then you can work out the best strategy for managing the condition together.

What to do in an asthma attack

The NHS Direct Healthcare Guide says that breathing difficulties in young children should never be ignored. If your child is wheezy and seems breathless you can call NHS Direct on 0845 4647 for advice, or dial 999 for an ambulance. Once your child has been diagnosed with asthma, you, your partner and any other carers like Granny or the babysitter should know what to do in the event of an asthma attack.

- Stay calm and reassure the child.
- Give him his reliever (blue) inhaler immediately, using a spacer if necessary.
- Don't put your arm round him, as this is constricting.
- Help him to breathe as slowly and calmly as possible while sitting in an upright position.

The medication should work in 5–10 minutes, leaving the child breathing normally again.

Call the doctor or an ambulance if

- the medication has no effect after 5–10 minutes;
- the child is extremely upset and unable to speak;
- the child seems exhausted;
- you have any doubts about his condition.

While you wait for help to arrive, continue to give the child medication – one 'puff' into a spacer every few minutes.

(For more detailed information about asthma medication, see Chapter 5.)

The GP's role

If your baby is wheezy or your toddler has repeated respiratory infections, both you and your GP might suspect asthma, especially if there is a family history. You have to remember that there is no single test that can be done that will give you a clear and immediate diagnosis. Dr Joe Neary of the Royal College of General Practitioners says that 10–15 per cent of GPs' time is spent dealing with respiratory problems, of which the most important is asthma.

We look after asthmatic children much better than we used to, and the majority of GP practices now have an asthma clinic, often run by a specially trained nurse. If your GP practice doesn't have such a clinic you might consider changing to one which does. These clinics focus on asthma alone. Your local Primary Care Trust or Health Authority will be able to tell you which practices in your area run asthma clinics.

It's very important to treat childhood asthma correctly because if we get it right in childhood, we very much reduce the risk of long-term lung damage.

Parents can help with the diagnosis by charting the child's symptoms over time as objectively and coolly as possible. Your GP will want to know

- if there is asthma or another allergic disease in the family;
- what the child's symptoms are – is he coughing a lot? Breathless? Is he wheezing? Is there any fever?
- whether the child's symptoms keep recurring;
- whether the symptoms are worse at any particular time (e.g. at night) or in particular circumstances (e.g. during exercise).

It's not always easy for the GP to decide whether your child has asthma, since other conditions may cause the same symptoms. Some children with asthma wheeze, others don't and coughing is their main symptom. However, it's important to get the diagnosis right, since under-treated asthma can often lead to children needing hospital care, and poorly controlled asthma can lead to other problems like stunted growth. So do continue to go to your GP when your child has respiratory infections, even if you haven't been given a definite diagnosis.

'Conditions other than asthma which also cause wheeze can be very frightening for both parents and children,' says Dr Neary.

Bronchiolitis, which typically affects children in their first year of life, leads to fever, distress, coughing and wheezing, but it is a viral infection and not asthma. Typically, a child who has had bronchiolitis will wheeze when he or she catches a cold, but two out of three wheezy pre-schoolers will stop wheezing by the time they get to school age.

It's worth remembering, too, that if you take your child to the doctor with a respiratory infection, you shouldn't assume that she will be given antibiotics.

'Antibiotics don't work against viral infections, or against asthma, so they are not appropriate treatments for wheezy babies and toddlers,' says Dr Neary.

The treatments that work best for asthmatic children are the range of preventers and relievers which are inhaled, either in the form of a spray or a dry powder. I would prescribe one of these according to the patient's preference.

The first step would be a reliever which the child could use whenever he experienced symptoms. If the asthma is mild and he only needs to use the reliever once or twice a week, that may be all the treatment that's needed. Understanding how the medication works and how to use the inhaler is very important too. Relievers should relieve symptoms in 20 minutes providing the inhaler has been used correctly. If standard asthma treatment like this doesn't seem to be working, and your child still wheezes significantly, has to stay at home from school, and can't sleep at night, then you should return to your GP who will look at the medication again.

Dr Neary says there are lots of 'mights' and 'maybes' in asthma treatment and there is no one-size-fits-all answer to some of the questions parents ask, like 'Should my child be referred to a specialist?' As he says,

If reliever medication doesn't seem to be working, your GP will suggest more robust treatment for the underlying problem, which means a 'preventer' in the form of a steroid spray. Parents are often wary of steroids but we know that a low-dose inhaler directed on the target has no adverse effects on growing children. It's only if the child's asthma does not respond to this kind of treatment and higher doses seem to be needed that a child may be referred for specialist help.

The right GP

Having the right GP can make all the difference, as Marie has found. Her son Stevie, 11, had his first asthma attack as a toddler.

Stevie had had a bad cold and then started wheezing so we called the doctor. Our GP takes a special interest in asthma and made me feel that it was something we could cope with, right from the start. He arrived with medication, a spacer and mask so that Stevie was treated straight away, and asked me to go into the surgery the next morning where I was given both preventer and reliever inhalers. Although Stevie was only little, he was never frightened of the treatment and got used to his inhalers really quickly. The doctor always explained to him what was happening, as well as me!

By the time he went to school he didn't need to use the mask any more and by the time he was 7 or 8 the doctor had showed him how to use his Ventolin inhaler by itself. Sport has always been a trigger for him but he soon learned to sit out if he was breathless or his chest felt tight, and take a puff or two of his inhaler.

More recently the doctor has prescribed a different inhaler which is a preventer and reliever in one and works more slowly. He just takes a puff of that morning and evening now and hardly ever needs to use his Ventolin. I'm not sure if Stevie is growing out of his asthma or if it's just that the current medication suits him, but our GP has been great every step of the way. My advice to parents would be to find a sympathetic GP. If yours isn't, ask for a second opinion or change doctors.

The asthma clinic

Most cases of childhood asthma are dealt with by GPs, often through a local asthma clinic attached to the practice. Only if the child doesn't seem to be responding to his medication or there are complications will he be referred on to a specialist. Children whose asthma is well controlled, who are confident about using the prescribed inhaler, and who are not having to take time off school or having sleepless nights because of asthma will probably only be asked to attend a couple of times a year. Children with more persistent symptoms whose asthma seems less well controlled will be asked to attend more often. Asthma experts stress that if you are using the medication as directed and it really doesn't seem to be helping, you should go back to your GP or asthma clinic and ask for a review. Medication is generally effective at controlling asthma, but it can take time for GPs and nurses to find exactly the right levels for your child.

What happens at the clinic?

A visit to an asthma clinic will include a 'peak flow test', when children are asked to breathe out as hard as they can into a tube called a 'peak flow meter' to measure how well their lungs are functioning. The correct peak flow levels in a healthy person have been worked out by height, age and sex, and usually the best of three readings is taken. These tests are usually quite popular with children, who like to see a high score! If your child's asthma seems unstable she may be asked to keep a peak flow diary, using the peak flow meter to check her own levels twice or possibly three times a day, at home, and making notes in the diary. In this way, the nurses can tell how well the medication is controlling her asthma and what adjustments might have to be made.

All the various inhalers, spacer and other devices will be there so that you can be shown how to use them effectively and, if necessary, choose a different type if you haven't been getting on with the one originally prescribed.

More comprehensive lung function tests are sometimes available but are not often needed for childhood asthma patients.

Your GP and the clinic staff all agree that the aim of the treatment is to enable your child to do everything his siblings and schoolmates do. With proper asthma management he should be symptom-free. If he isn't, it could be back to the drawing-board until his asthma is under control.

For more detailed information about the medication used to control asthma, see Chapter 5.

Unless your child's asthma is very severe, you will be seeing more of your GP and asthma nurse than any other member of the medical profession so it helps if you get on well.

'Most GPs try very hard to help their patients and are very knowledgeable,' says Dr Neary.

However, some are better at listening and communicating than others. Parents of asthmatic children can help by trying to stay calm and reasonable even when they are worried about the child's health. GPs can help by reassuring patients that they are welcome to come back – indeed, they *should* come back – if the medication does not seem to be working. That way, the family all feel that the problem is being taken seriously. If there is a personality clash or you really don't feel that your GP is listening to your concerns, you should consider finding another GP. This isn't an admission of failure – someone else might simply be better able to help you and your child.

If your child has an acute attack: A&E

In 2002 the National Asthma Campaign Scotland produced a report, *Sleepless Nights, Anxious Days*, looking at the everyday problems faced by parents with asthmatic children. Many said that having to take their child to A&E with an acute asthma attack was among the most traumatic experiences they had to face. A busy Accident and Emergency department is, of course, not the most friendly or hospitable of places for children. The staff have to deal with a wide variety of patients with all sorts of medical and social problems at all hours of the day and night.

It has been recommended that all A&E departments have a children-only area and two specialist paediatric nurses on duty all the time, but staff shortages sometimes mean that this is not the case. Parents have complained that they have to answer the same questions over and over, that they are not always able to see a respiratory specialist and that it can take far too long for a sick child to be admitted to a children's ward.

'We have seen quite dramatic changes in the way children are treated in A&E in the last few years,' says Dr John Heyworth of the British Association for Accident and Emergency Medicine.

I wouldn't claim that everything is perfect, but treatment is getting better. Traditionally, in the old casualty departments, children were just dumped in with adults but these days there is usually a special paediatric area in the department, staffed by nurses who have experience in working with children.

Again, until recently, children who came to A&E tended to be seen by quite junior doctors but now they are seen by senior nurses and doctors.

Children who are suffering from acute asthma attacks should be in a properly equipped and staffed A&E environment, and concerned parents shouldn't hesitate to bring their child in if he is not responding to his usual medication. At the hospital where I work, our children's A&E employs distraction techniques like light displays, bubbles and play specialists. The picture for children in A&E has changed and is still changing, including much better liaison with the paediatric departments of hospitals.

How can parents help, when their child has to go into A&E with an acute asthma attack?

'The rate of deterioration in children can be quite dramatic so parents shouldn't hesitate to bring them in as soon as there is a problem,' says Dr Heyworth. 'Many can be treated with a nebulizer and are soon well enough to go home. If they're not we keep them under observation and then admit them to the children's ward if necessary.'

Parents should bring the child's current medication with them, or at least know what it is. They should be able to tell the medical staff:

- how long the child has been breathless or wheezing;
- if the problem has been building up gradually, or came on suddenly;
- what treatment the child has been given;
- if this has happened before and what the outcome was – for instance, did the child have to be admitted to a high-dependency bed or intensive care?
- if the child has any other illnesses or is on other medication.

'A child will usually be discharged once his condition has stabilized, but parents know their child best. If, after treatment in A&E, he still doesn't seem himself, the parents should tell the doctors so,' says Dr Heyworth.

It's important to remember that most children with asthma never need to go to A&E at all. It's only the minority who don't respond to standard treatment from their GP or asthma clinic, and whose asthma is difficult to control, who end up in an A&E department.

Denise, whose teenage son Josh has severe asthma, says that the treatment he gets in the children's A&E department at her local hospital is brilliant now, but that that wasn't always the case.

When I first took him to A&E I didn't know much about asthma treatment and they just used to nebulize him and send him home, without suggesting a follow-up appointment or anything. The trouble is that A&E doctors aren't asthma experts. One told me that steroid drugs always worked for asthmatic children when I knew that Josh is one of the minority who don't respond well to them. I think they just thought I was a pushy parent! But over the years it has got much better, and if we have to go to A&E, I now say what treatment Josh should have. If he is really ill he goes straight up to the ward without having to wait. At my GP's surgery it's the same, he is seen straight away.

Doctors could help by explaining what all the tests and readings are for and parents should learn as much as possible about treatments and what they do.

The British Thoracic Society guidelines

The British Thoracic Society's most recent guidelines on the management of childhood asthma in A&E departments point out that if children have to attend A&E, especially on a regular basis, it's a sign that their asthma medication isn't working as it should. It should, therefore, be reviewed. They recommend that A&E staff:

- check the child's inhaler technique;
- consider the need for inhaled steroids to be prescribed (i.e. preventer as well as reliever medication);
- provide a written asthma plan in case of subsequent attacks;
- arrange follow-up by the patient's GP within a week;
- arrange follow-up in a children's asthma clinic within 1–2 months.

Communication is really the key to a good relationship with the medical staff looking after your child, from GPs to asthma nurses and specialists. They may be the experts when it comes to treating asthma, but you know more than they do about your child and, as you're with him all the time, you are often best placed to say whether his condition is getting worse or better, and how well he is coping with his medication. Never be afraid to ask questions if there's something you don't understand. It often helps to jot down your questions before you go into the surgery or clinic – and take notes while you are there.

5

Managing Asthma

With today's effective treatments, it should be possible for all but a very small minority of asthmatic children to lead normal lives – going to school, meeting friends, taking part in sports and games, going on holiday, and enjoying everything that other children enjoy. If asthma can't yet be cured, it can usually be controlled with a combination of drug treatments and perhaps some minor adjustments to family lifestyle.

As we've already seen, it is quite difficult to diagnose asthma in very young children. There are many other conditions which can cause wheezing in a baby or toddler. Once your child has been diagnosed with asthma, however, it's important that the condition be brought under control as soon as it's practically possible.

Preventers and relievers

There are two main kinds of medicines used to treat asthma. They are known as **preventers** and **relievers**. These involve quite different drugs and work in different ways. Both are, however, usually **inhaled**, simply because this delivers the medication straight to the lungs where it is most effective.

Preventers normally come in brown, white, orange or red inhalers and are usually (though not always) corticosteroid drugs like beclomethasone (Becotide and Becloforte), budesonide (Pulmicort) and fluticasone (Flixotide). Corticosteroids are synthetic copies of the natural hormones produced by the body. They act by reducing inflammation, so when breathed in they help to calm swollen and highly sensitive airways, which are then less likely to flare up when they come across an asthma trigger. Preventers reduce the risk of severe asthma attacks and their effectiveness builds up over a period of time, usually about five days. If your child is prescribed preventer medication, she will be advised to take it twice a day, even when she is symptom-free. Another kind of preventer is sodium cromoglycate (Intal, Cromogen) which is not a steroid. It has to be taken regularly, up to four times a day, and also before exercise. This is not always convenient for school-age children whose parents aren't around to remind them to take their medication regularly! It may also take several weeks of regular medication to produce an effect. It is sometimes prescribed for children with mild to moderate asthma whose parents really don't like the idea of them taking steroids.

About steroids

The steroids prescribed as asthma preventers are not to be confused with the anabolic steroids used in body-building, and they have a good safety record. Parents are naturally concerned about the idea of long-term steroid use in young children. However, the fact that in most cases steroids are inhaled means that very little of the drug is absorbed by the rest of the body, and side-effects are extremely rare. Your GP will prescribe the lowest possible dose of steroids necessary to keep your child's asthma under control. Research studies have shown that children using inhaled steroids do tend to grow slightly more slowly than children who don't take them, but they go on growing for longer so they attain the same height by the time they are adults.

For instance, a four-year study of 3,347 children with asthma on Tayside in Scotland in 1998 found that neither asthma nor treatments for asthma had any appreciable effect on the growth rates of most of the children. Social deprivation affected children's height and weight much more than asthma did. However, the minority of children whose asthma was severe enough for them to be on high doses of inhaled steroids, and who were frequently admitted to hospital because of their asthma, were shorter and lighter than the other children in the study.

For the minority of children whose asthma cannot be controlled by inhaled steroids and who need to take tablets, side-effects may be more of a problem. For instance, they can occasionally cause growth problems, acne and mood swings, and lead to a child putting on weight. This is why your child's asthma treatment needs to be carefully monitored. Steroid tablets can also lower the body's resistance to chicken pox, so if your child has been in contact with this illness while on steroids it's wise to consult your GP.

Bronchodilators
Relievers are the medicines that your child takes as soon as asthma symptoms come on. As the name suggests, they relieve the unpleasant symptoms of wheezing, coughing and breathlessness. Reliever drugs are known as bronchodilators. They work by relaxing

the muscles surrounding the bronchioles – the narrow air passages within the lungs. They are effective within a few minutes and the effect lasts for up to four hours. Reliever medication comes in the familiar blue inhalers that asthmatic children carry around with them. Well-known bronchodilators include salbutamol (Ventolin) and terbutaline (Bricanyl). Ipratropium bromide (Atrovent) is a different kind of bronchodilator which tends to act more slowly but lasts longer. It works in a similar way to the others, and is most often prescribed for very small children as salbutamol is sometimes less effective in treating this age group. Salbutamol syrup can be prescribed for very small children, or they can be prescribed anti-histamines instead. Side-effects from these medicines are usually minimal, though they can make children a little hyperactive. In exceptionally severe cases, reliever drugs like terbutaline can be delivered by means of a 24-hour pump.

There are also more long-lasting drugs, modified bronchodilators like salmeterol and eformoterol, which are designed to stay in the airways for a longer period. They are usually in green inhalers, and work over about 12 hours to keep the airways relaxed. Brand names include Serevent and Oxis. They are usually prescribed in more severe cases, perhaps when a child has not really responded to the more usual combination of an inhaled steroid as a preventer, with a reliever when needed.

Inhalers, spacers, masks and nebulizers

Seeing the variety of differently coloured and shaped inhalers plus spacers, masks and nebulizers can be very confusing at first for both parents and children. They have names like 'Turbohaler' and 'Autohaler' and 'Easy-Breathe' but the job they do is basically the same – delivering an appropriate dose of medication to your child's airways and lungs. It is obviously vital that your child has an inhaler that he can easily use and which both he and you feel happy and comfortable with. This means that you need to take some time with your GP or asthma nurse to find out exactly how to use the inhaler you have been prescribed.

'Inhalers come in so many shapes and sizes and some are more effective in delivering medication than others, depending on the age and ability of the child,' says asthma nurse Liz Biggart.

Having so many devices to choose from means that it is now possible to deliver inhaled medication effectively, even to toddlers. Parents and children need to be shown how to use their inhaler so that they feel totally confident about using it and don't feel frightened or silly.

Very small children and babies under about 2 years old will need a spacer and a mask as well as the inhaler, because they can't co-ordinate their breathing as older children can.

A spacer is a clear plastic device looking rather like a water-bottle with a mouthpiece at one end and, if required, a mask that fits over the child's face. The inhaler is attached to the other end and medication is puffed in for the child to breathe. Spacers make inhalers easier for young children to use, and are more effective at delivering the right amount of medication than inhalers on their own.

'A mask can look frightening at first so I encourage mums and toddlers to play with it before they try to use it,' Liz says.

You can stick little pictures on to the spacer to make it more child-friendly, and play games like 'Peep-Bo' with it. You can put it over Mum's face or the nurse's face first so that the child gets used to seeing it.

Give your child plenty of cuddles and praise when she holds it over her own mouth for a few seconds. Tell her it will make her feel better. Take it slowly, and choose a time to introduce it when the child isn't exhausted or busy. Hold the child, cuddle her, sing to her, tell her a story or let her watch a video while she uses it.

We find that even really small children soon learn to ask for their mask if they are feeling wheezy, once they know it makes them feel better. Parents should also tell their toddlers that they might have to put on their mask if they cough in the night, because if they wake up and find they have a mask on they may be frightened.

Young children with very severe asthma might have to use a nebulizer. This is a machine which turns medication into a fine mist which is easy for even the smallest children to inhale. As other devices like inhalers and spacers are developed, there is less and less need for children to use nebulizers, but if your child's doctors feel that he needs one you will be shown how to use it.

It's really important to make sure that your child learns to use his inhaler happily and effectively so it's worth persevering and making sure you get it right! Doctors and asthma nurses are happy to give you as much time as you need to get used to an inhaler and spacer. Once you have got used to it, it's yours for life or as long as the child's asthma lasts, so make sure you feel happy with the inhaler your child uses. From about the age of 5 your child might be sufficiently co-ordinated to use an inhaler without a spacer. He will be asked to shake the inhaler, then sigh out, then breathe in, using the inhaler, for a count of ten.

Some doctors like to prescribe combined asthma medication, consisting of steroid drugs like fluticasone, as a preventer, plus salmeterol, a long-acting reliever, which reduces the number of doses a child needs.

'Whichever type of inhaler or spacer you use, it's always important to be taught properly and be sure your child is getting the most out of it,' says asthma nurse Liz Biggart.

The drug companies which make anti-asthma drugs also make inhalers so you need to use the appropriate inhaler for a particular drug. Once you have chosen a suitable inhaler and learned how to use it then you should always use that type. Make using the inhaler a regular habit like brushing teeth, so that it involves minimal effort and you don't even have to think about it. Perhaps it could be kept next to the child's toothbrush. It should certainly be kept where the child can see it so that she remembers to use her preventer, even when she's feeling well. If a child's asthma is mild she can afford to miss the occasional dose without any real ill-effects, but it's much better to get into regular habits or the asthma is likely to get worse.

Denise's son Josh has severe asthma and has used different inhalers over the years. She says that it's important for parents to realize that many different types are available and that if your child has difficulty using one, another may be more suitable.

Josh always found breath-activated ones like the Acuhaler difficult to use because he never had enough breath to make them work. However, the 'push-down' types like Ventolin seemed to work well for him and he was able to manage his inhaler plus spacer by himself from his first year at primary school. He doesn't mind the taste, and finds that he doesn't suffer from sore throats and hoarseness, which can happen with some inhalers.

I would advise parents to have a chat to a specialist asthma nurse who will be able to show them all the different kinds of inhalers you can get. At first I just wasn't aware how much choice there is, but nurses keep up to date with new models on the market. Sometimes it's easier to talk to a nurse than a doctor, as well.

Asthma and family life

Managing asthma is really about

- getting a correct diagnosis;
- being prescribed the right medication;
- using the medication as directed;

but that isn't the whole story. Many parents ask if their family life has to change because they have a child with asthma, but asthma experts say that exposure to a normal environment is best for children's health.

'You can't keep your child in a sterile bubble, and your goal should be to enable him or her to lead a normal life, doing normal things,' says Liz Biggart.

Asthma is an individual condition and no two cases are exactly the same, but it can be predictable for an individual. Parents learn to understand how asthma affects their child, and work around that. Parents observe what triggers off an asthma attack and they can then work out how to avoid the worst triggers [see Chapter 3]. You don't have to tear your home apart; simple housekeeping strategies like buying new pillows and washing bed-linen at 60° can be a real help, as can making sure your home is well ventilated.

Not all doctors agree that allergen avoidance is useful, or even practical.

'The one thing that we know is a problem for children with asthma is house-dust mite,' says Dr Neary of the Royal College of GPs.

There are various methods of controlling house-dust mites in the home, like using mite-proof covers on mattresses, washing bed-linen at high temperatures or with special detergents, vacuuming with special cleaners, and so on. Children will undoubtedly benefit from a reduction in the number of house-dust mites but it can be very difficult to sustain. In clinical terms, reducing the level of mites a little will not achieve very much although it may be comforting! Dusting and vacuuming may just spread the problem around and house-dust mites breed so quickly you could be fighting a losing battle against them. There must be laboratories somewhere working on a method of stopping them from breeding, but if they have come up with a solution I have yet to hear of it!

Linda's 13-year-old son Nicholas has very severe asthma and she says it has taken its toll on their family life. He is now under the care of the specialist asthma clinic at the Royal Brompton Hospital in London as he has been having bad asthma attacks every two weeks.

'We haven't really been able to do anything as a family for the last three or four years,' Linda says.

We can't make plans to go out or go on holiday. My family live on the South Coast and we just can't go and visit them. Nick has only managed two hours a day in school, which is very isolating for him. He worries a lot because his asthma attacks are very frightening, but anxiety can make them worse. He has ended up in our local hospital eight or nine times in the last year. Since last winter we have had instant access to the chest ward at our local hospital when Nick has a severe attack.

We haven't really been able to find out what triggers off his asthma. He did have a RAST test – a blood test which is designed to identify particular allergies as well as find out how allergic a child is. The results indicated that house-dust mites were a problem for him, so we bought some special allergy-proof bedding and a Dyson vacuum cleaner with a HEPA filter. I vacuum the bed and the carpets and the rest of the furniture regularly but I'm not sure whether it has made any difference. Sometimes going out in cold weather seemed to bring on an attack; on another occasion he visited a friend who had had a dog in the house – even though the dog wasn't there – but it's never immediately obvious what is causing the attacks.

We're a strong family and we do try to think positive. In a way, it doesn't help that so many children these days have asthma, because people tend to say oh, yeah, asthma, you have to use an inhaler, okay – but it can be more serious than that.

Most parents, like Linda, find asthma worrying, especially if their child is severely affected. The NAC's recent report, *Sleepless Nights, Anxious Days*, found that asthma did have an impact on family lifestyles. A quarter of the parents surveyed were woken one or more times a week because of the child's asthma, and one in six had had to take time off work. Perhaps the most common difficulty described by the parents interviewed for this book was the constant anxiety. Parents are always concerned that their child may have an asthma attack – particularly when he is away from home – yet they recognize that children need more independence as they get older.

As single mum Donna says,

You do worry, yet you don't want to treat your child differently from other children or make her stand out from the rest. I try very hard not to over-protect Julie. Communication is the answer. I make sure that everyone knows she has an inhaler so that when she is at school or going out with family friends, they know that she may need a couple of puffs if she gets breathless. I've never stopped her doing what all the other kids do, though I have had a few anxious moments!

Specialist suppliers' catalogues and literature from the National Asthma Campaign and Allergy UK will list many products which claim to cut down on allergens, from air purifiers to vacuum cleaners with special filters, pet wipes to special bedding. How can you know whether these products will help your child? Most experts agree that it's worth trying the cheaper options first – like making sure your home is well ventilated and airing the bed before you make it up – before you spend a lot of money on specialist equipment.

The NAC, for instance, can't endorse particular products because there is rarely any scientific evidence that one product is better than another of the same type.

The Consumers' Association, through its magazines *Which?* and *Health Which?*, does sometimes review useful products and produce objective reports on which ones seem to work best. Contact the CA (address on p. 80) for details of recent tests.

Medical evidence suggests that vacuuming regularly with an efficient vacuum cleaner does help to clear allergens from your home. Upright cleaners are said to be slightly better at this than cylinders. You can also buy cleaners with HEPA filters, which are said to be more effective, though one *Which?* report in the late 1990s cast doubt on this.

Since the majority of asthmatic children are sensitive to house-dust mites, mite-proof bedding would seem a sensible option. House-dust mites are said to be able to colonize a new mattress within four months! Department stores and mail-order companies like The Healthy House (address on p. 80) stock these, and both the NAC and *Health Which?* have found that most leading brands were equally effective. The best type of cover is one which fits over the whole mattress rather than just the top. It should also be a 'breathable' fabric which feels comfortable and should suit your budget. It's also a matter of personal choice whether you use feather or synthetic pillows. If your child is allergic to feathers, obviously synthetics are a better choice. Mite-proof pillow covers are also available. Ionizers and air filters are of doubtful benefit in reducing allergens, and ionizers may actually make symptoms worse.

The NAC points out that, quite often, the simplest and cheapest methods of allergen reduction, like keeping your home well ventilated and dusting with a damp cloth, are among the most effective. Before you spend a lot of money on special products, contact them (details on p. 78) for the most up-to-date advice.

A word about holidays

Once your child's asthma is well controlled by medication, there's no reason why you shouldn't go away on family holidays like everyone else. Mention holiday plans to your GP or asthma nurse and take a few extra precautions when you are packing.

Don't forget to take your child's inhaler, plus any tablets he needs. Take a spare and enough medication for a few extra days in case of airport hold-ups or other emergencies.

Don't let the change in routine make your child forget his regular treatment. Even if he's feeling perfectly well and dying to get to the beach or the pool, he should take his preventer medication as usual. You might mention to the holiday rep that your child has asthma and find out the name of a local doctor or the arrangements for taking your child to a health centre or hospital in an emergency.

When taking out medical insurance for your holiday, make sure you tell the insurers that your child has asthma. Some policies exclude 'pre-existing medical conditions' so you need to be absolutely sure that you are covered. Remember, you don't have to take out the insurance offered by the holiday company. Shopping around may get you a better deal. If you are travelling within the

EU, don't forget your Form E111, obtainable from the Post Office as part of the *Health Advice for Travellers* booklet. This entitles you to medical treatment in EU countries on the same terms as the locals. But be warned: you may have to pay for treatment and then claim some or all of the money back afterwards, so be sure to keep all receipts.

If you are flying, make sure you carry any inhalers in your hand luggage. Many airlines have banned smoking, but if you fly with one that hasn't done so, be sure your family sit as far away from the smoking section as possible.

If you use dust mite-proof bedding on your child's mattress and pillow at home, take them with you.

If you plan a camping holiday, think about how your child reacts to pollen.

According to the NAC, house-dust mites can't live above the snow-line, so a skiing holiday might be a good idea. However, this doesn't apply if your child's asthma is triggered by very cold weather.

For children severely affected by asthma, the NAC organizes special supervised activity holidays. They are aimed at children aged 6–12 and also young people aged 12–17, and are often based in boarding-school premises in different parts of the UK. They are staffed by trained volunteers and health professionals, with GP and hospital expertise nearby if required.

'Most of the children who come on PEAK holidays are those whose asthma affects their quality of life,' says holidays manager Patrick Ladbury.

It may be moderate or severe or they may have additional problems like eczema or food allergies which make it difficult for them to go on normal school trips. Some may have been bullied at school and dislike being made to feel 'different'.

As well as ordinary fun activities like swimming, treasure hunts and visits to theme parks, we offer asthma-related educational activities, so that the children are able to learn more about asthma management. This is especially valuable for teenage participants, who are encouraged to be independent and start to take care of themselves, taking control of their own asthma and learning to recognize their own symptoms.

The children enjoy meeting others with the same condition, sometimes for the first time. The holidays can increase their self-confidence as they are able to do things they never thought they could do. Many of the volunteers have asthma as well so there are role models for them. Sometimes children with asthma are rather over-protected at home. Being on holiday shows them they can do things by themselves. It also gives their parents a break, a chance for them to be a couple or give more time to brothers and sisters – or re-decorate or spring-clean, which is difficult to do with an asthmatic child in the house!

We have also just started to do 'family weekends' for parents with children aged up to 10.

PEAK holidays usually last a week and are very reasonably priced, with parents being asked for a contribution according to their means.

You can find out more by contacting the PEAK manager at the NAC (address on p. 78).

Laura's 12-year-old son has been on two PEAK holidays and she says the benefits have been remarkable, not only for her son but for her as well.

'Before Ben went on the PEAK holiday I never felt I could let him out of my sight,' she admits. 'Now, he goes to the local park with his friends and I feel okay about it. Those holidays have done as much for me as they have for Ben!'

Laura is a single parent and Ben has very severe asthma. He has been in and out of hospital ever since he was born. Laura helped to run a support group for children with asthma and their families, but even though she had seen other children grow in confidence after their holidays, it was hard for her to 'hand her precious son over to strangers'!

I must have driven them mad. I was a nervous wreck letting him go, but he came back totally euphoric. Ben was quite an introverted little boy who felt self-conscious about using his inhaler in front of other people. The PEAK holidays taught him that it was okay to be 'different' and he had the time of his life. He had joined the Scouts but had had to miss out on a lot of activities. When he went on the PEAK holiday, they asked him what he had always wanted to do. He said he had always wanted to sleep in a tent, with a torch, so that was what he did. Even if he never does it again at least he knows what it's like. He was also put in charge of a younger child, which he thought was fantastic. Being with other children who had similar medical problems helped him to feel comfortable and accept his condition. Ben told me afterwards he felt it was the first time he hadn't had to prove himself. It gave him the chance to push his boundaries out and do things in a safe, supervised setting.

As for me, I knew I could trust the staff to look after him. I had never really felt like that about anyone else. His father takes him on holiday but I can never relax while they're away. My sister is a nurse and I even felt nervous leaving Ben with her! At the same time, I knew I had to learn to let Ben go, and this was a safe way to do it. When you have a severely asthmatic child, you're a nurse as well as a mum. We start every day with the same routine of inhalers and nasal sprays and anti-histamines. I always have to check that the medication isn't running out. My life has pretty much revolved round Ben's asthma ever since he was born. For the week he went on the holiday, I felt I could take a real break as well.

The NAC regularly gets thank-you letters from young holiday-makers. Lorna's is typical.

I am writing to say that I had a wonderful time. It was great fun, I met loads of friends, and best of all, I didn't have to worry about anything to do with my eczema or asthma. At first I didn't want to go on the holiday as I am very shy, but I was really glad that I went.

6

What Carers, Childminders and Teachers Should Know

Parents and children soon get used to managing asthma symptoms at home and avoiding, as far as possible, the triggers that could lead to an asthma attack. But what happens when your child is old enough for playgroup or school? It's not easy finding the right child care for small children, especially those with asthma. Whether your pre-school child is cared for by a family member, a childminder or nanny, it's obviously vital that the carer knows as much as possible about the child's asthma. When care is shared – for instance, if your toddler goes to playgroup or nursery school for part of the time – everyone involved should be equally well informed. Babysitters should also be aware that your child has asthma, should know what symptoms to look out for and what to do if your child has an asthma attack.

Pre-school care

Good communication is the key here, as is proper preparation. When you are looking for a childminder or other carer, you will need to ask the same questions every parent asks. You want to be sure your child will be happy and well cared for. Naturally, you will want to know that the nursery or minder is properly registered with the Local Authority, and that they have your contact numbers so that you can be reached in an emergency. With an asthmatic child, there are other checks to be made, for instance:

- Will anyone be smoking around him at any time?
- Are there pets in the home or nursery which might trigger an asthma attack?
- Do carers know exactly how and when to use your child's medication?
- Would they be able to recognize and deal with an emergency, such as a severe asthma attack?

The National Asthma Campaign (address on p. 78) has useful information about this, including a leaflet on policy guidelines for pre-school groups, covering the different kinds of pre-school providers like nurseries and playgroups. The leaflet makes the point that staff should be trained to deal with children with asthma so that they feel confident about helping these very little ones to use their inhaler, including the use of a spacer if necessary. Everyone involved, including the child, should know where the inhaler is kept and it should be readily accessible if needed. The NAC produces two cards, a school card and an asthma management plan card, which can help parents and nurseries to work together to manage a child's asthma.

If your child is cared for by a childminder, it is reassuring to know that the National Childminding Association has guidelines which cover the use of any kind of medication. They suggest that you discuss it with your childminder so that she understands what is needed. Written records have to be kept by the childminder with details of any medication she has given to your child, plus times and dosages. This record has to be signed by minders and parents.

The Pre-School Learning Alliance (address on p. 81) publishes *The Accident Prevention Book* which has information about health and safety issues for young children. Among the guidelines is information about children who have asthma. This includes a brief description of the condition and a guide to what to do if a child has an asthma attack. The Alliance points out that very young children should carry their own anti-asthma medication with them and recommends that staff and parents sit down together to discuss the child's condition and treatment.

It is now felt that children with asthma shouldn't be excluded from playgroups, nurseries, or the same range of early-learning experiences that other children have, unless it's absolutely necessary. Although little ones may become wheezy during exercise either indoors or out, a puff of their reliever medication beforehand should enable them to run around with the other children. If the playgroup wants to include the experience of looking after pets, stick insects, fish or perhaps a tortoise might be more suitable than hamsters, guinea-pigs or gerbils. In the rare cases where a child's asthma is triggered by an allergy to a particular foodstuff such as egg, it might be possible for cookery lessons to exclude this.

Again, written records of the medication a child has been prescribed should be kept. The Alliance recommends that

- any medication must have been prescribed by a doctor;
- all medication should be in its original packaging;

- dosage and timing should match the instructions on the pack;
- staff should be trained how to use it if necessary;
- parents should have agreed to the timing and dosage;
- a child's inhaler should be given to his key worker and kept in a safe accessible place, so that both know where it is.

The Anaphylaxis Campaign (address on p. 79) has also issued guidelines for carers of pre-school children.

At school

In recent years, and especially with the rise in the numbers of children with asthmatic symptoms, it has been recognized that chronic conditions like asthma can be successfully managed within an ordinary school environment. In 1996, the Department for Education and Skills and the Department of Health issued a booklet called *Supporting Children with Medical Needs*. This aimed to help schools draw up guidelines, ensuring that pupils with conditions like asthma could be accommodated in all schools. Asthma nurse Liż Biggart says that there has been a change in teachers' attitudes to asthmatic pupils in the last ten years anyway.

> There is much more awareness of pupils' needs. In the past, staff attitudes tended to be that they were there to teach, and that what happened in their pupils' lives beyond the school gates was not their problem. However, since the various directives from the Department, teachers have been more likely to say that they will help to make sure asthmatic children don't miss out on education.
> It is really up to parents and health professionals to make sure that heads and teachers know what is needed.

Mollie is the head of a small inner-city infants' school catering for children between 4 and 7 years old.

> We only have two children with asthma this year, an unusually small number for us. Normally, in our school there will be five or six. Because the children are so little, we keep the inhalers locked up in my office and the children come up every lunchtime for their medication, which is always supervised by the same welfare assistant, or by myself if she isn't there. The parents have to inform us in writing of exactly what medication the child has and

give us permission to supervise their child. They also let us know if there are any changes and we keep in close touch if the medication is running out.

When I was an assistant teacher at another school a child in my class had a severe asthma attack on his second day in school. It was extremely frightening as his mother had promised to bring his inhaler but had not yet done so. There was nothing I could do except dial 999. When the ambulance arrived the paramedic gave him oxygen and I went with him to A&E and stayed with him till we managed to contact his parents.

That was ten years ago, when asthma was less well catered for in schools. These days, there are so many children with medical conditions. As well as asthmatics I have two with anaphylaxis and one diabetic.

Both the DES guidelines and a leaflet from the National Union of Teachers explain what asthma is and how school pupils can be helped to manage the condition while causing as little disruption as possible to their ordinary school life. Again, good communication is the key. As the parent of an asthmatic child you should be sure that the head teacher, your child's class teacher, form tutor, head of year and anyone with responsibility for him should know that he has asthma, what his treatment consists of, and which factors are likely to trigger an attack. Depending on the circumstances in individual schools, other staff might also need to know – classroom and playground assistants, sports staff and supply teachers, for instance. You might suggest that, if it's appropriate in your child's case,

- any pets are removed from the classroom;
- care should be taken with fumes when working in a science lab;
- care should be taken over ingredients/materials in cookery, art or woodwork classes;
- staff should keep an eye on your child if the pollen count is high or the weather especially cold;
- your child should not be forced to play games if she feels wheezy or uncomfortable.

This is *not*, however, an excuse for children to avoid any exercise, which is as essential for children with asthma as it is for other children. Children who keep fit with regular exercise are less likely to be troubled by their asthma. 'Warming up' gently before exercise can sometimes help. A couple of puffs of reliever medication before

PE and games lessons should enable your child to take part in normal school sports and activities. If it doesn't, contact your GP or asthma nurse, as it is likely that his medication needs to be adjusted. Remember that top sports stars like marathon runner Paula Radcliffe and Manchester United and England soccer star Paul Scholes both have asthma!

Schools' asthma policies

Schools have their own policies on some aspects of asthma management. For example, not all schools allow younger children to carry their inhaler with them at all times, even though the DES guidelines state that schoolchildren should have 'immediate access to their reliever inhalers when they need them'.

This is something that parents, pupils and teachers need to work out between them. Quite often, the reason for the ban is that staff are afraid – or know only too well – that children are likely to lose their inhalers, or have them stolen, damaged or misused by other children. Children in primary schools may need help in taking their medication and there is also concern about other children taking a puff out of curiosity. However, healthcare professionals agree that it is unlikely that a child would come to any harm by doing this – though, obviously, it should be discouraged! It is suggested that parents provide a spare inhaler, in case the original is lost, left at home or runs out. Inhalers should always be marked with the pupil's name and stored in a safe place. Remember that inhalers have a 'use-by' date, and make sure that the one your child carries and the spare kept at school are not out of date.

If the school does not agree that your child should have her inhaler with her at all times, you should make sure that she knows where it is kept and that she is not too shy or embarrassed to ask her teacher if she feels she needs it. Inhalers should always be readily accessible whether your child is in the classroom, in the playground, or taking part in sport in a gym or on the playing field. Arrangements must also be made when there is a school trip or outing.

Jo is a class teacher in a suburban primary school. Among her class of 7–8-year-olds this year is one boy with asthma.

Our school policy is that all children with asthma should have access to their inhalers whenever they need them. This applies to children from 5 to 11. We have to balance this with not leaving them where other kids can mess about with them!

Jack's inhalers live in the top drawer of my desk, and he is allowed to go to my desk and get one whenever he thinks he needs it. He sees this as a bit of a perk as none of the other children are allowed to open my desk drawers for any reason! This has always worked fine and no child has ever abused this trust.

We have a board in the staffroom where we pin up details of which children in which class have medical conditions like asthma and diabetes, so that all the staff are informed. My classroom is never locked at lunchtime so if Jack had a bad attack he, or a dinner lady or another child in my class, could get in and fetch the inhaler. All the children in the class know where to find it and so do the dinner ladies.

Asthma is rather different from other medical conditions. If any of the children have to take pills, for example, they have to be kept in the office cupboard and given out by the welfare assistant. But keeping inhalers in the classroom is not a problem.

Asthma nurse Liz Biggart feels that children at secondary or middle schools are old enough to be allowed to keep their inhalers with them, especially given the size of some school campuses. She points out that a child who feels an attack of wheezing and breathlessness coming on is in no position to walk half a mile to find a teacher to collect the inhaler. A child or young teenager might also feel shy and self-conscious about knocking on the staffroom door. The National Asthma Campaign recommends that children be allowed to take responsibility for their inhaler from the age of about 7. If your child's school is unwilling for him to do this, or the school brushes aside your concerns, you might have to consider whether this is really the right school for your child.

The National Asthma Campaign has a Schools Pack which it can send out to any school which doesn't yet have an asthma policy. This includes information about the condition and the medication usually prescribed, a guide to what to do in an emergency, information about PE and sports, help for class teachers when an asthmatic child joins the class, and ways to increase awareness of asthma among school students. The NAC is currently campaigning for 'spare' inhalers to be kept in all schools for emergency use, as at the present time an inhaler can only be obtained by the person for whom it was prescribed.

Schools are not required by law to keep records of medication given to pupils but it is regarded as good practice for them to do so. Forms are available from the DES for schools to do this and your school may ask you, as a parent, to fill one in, detailing

- the name of your child's medication;
- dose;
- method of administration;
- time and frequency of administration;
- any side-effects.

Other forms give details of emergency contact numbers for you and your GP and an agreement to be signed if you want your child to be allowed to carry and administer her own medication. This all adds up to a 'Healthcare Plan' for your child at school and means that everyone knows exactly what their responsibilities are.

With so many asthmatic children in British schools these days it's easier than it once was to maintain a matter-of-fact attitude to the condition and the medication involved. However, some children are still teased and feel self-conscious if they have to use an inhaler and this is something that staff and parents should watch out for. All schools have anti-bullying policies but children who seem to be 'different' in some way can be easy targets. Nor are all teachers as sympathetic as they might be.

'Josh had a games teacher who wanted him to take part in cross-country runs when he really wasn't up to it,' said Josh's mother.

He kept saying 'your asthma can't be that bad' when, in fact, Josh is one of the minority of children whose asthma didn't respond well to inhaled steroids. He was then given tablets which caused side-effects such as weight gain and mood swings, as well as nose bleeds. I felt that his teachers weren't making allowances for the treatment he was on and treating him like a stroppy teenager rather than a child with health problems. The asthma clinic staff were very helpful, though, and offered to write a letter to the school explaining what the problem was. He wasn't trying to bunk off games, I just wish he could have been allowed to do something less strenuous than cross-country!

The west London borough of Hillingdon has a sophisticated asthma management strategy in its schools, based on a children's asthma group which incorporates the local hospital, GPs, paediatricians, pharmacists, the Education Authority and individual schools. Asthma nurse Alison Summerfield regularly goes into the 100 local schools to monitor their asthma policies and make sure they are actually working.

We started this about ten years ago when I was working with a young girl with very severe asthma. Her school really needed advice about how her condition was to be managed and I'm pleased to say that she managed to go through both primary and secondary schooling here without any problems.

I still find that parents are not always being given the right information when their child is diagnosed. Many don't really understand the difference between preventer and reliever medication. I have found some children in school still using a spacer with a mask, which is really only suitable for children up to the age of about 3. Their parents haven't been told that the condition needs to be regularly monitored. Some GPs have asthma clinics but parents are not told about them – so part of my job over the last ten years has been to educate health professionals, parents and schools, as well as children.

These days we expect all our schools to have an asthma policy in place and working. We recommend that schools have a register of children with asthma, and that each child should have at least one inhaler in school, and ideally two – one with the child at all times, and the other easily accessible in an emergency. All our schools now have a named asthma nurse. Our role is to offer ongoing support to staff and children, to review the cases of children who are having to miss school because of their asthma, and to run training courses for staff, so that they can update their skills.

It's important that children have access to reliever medication when they need it. If their asthma is properly controlled, they shouldn't need to use an inhaler often, but it should always be available, in the classroom.

Schools manage this in different ways. In primary schools, for example, many children need a spacer as well as an inhaler. Spacers are too big to fit in a child's pocket. Some schools have spacers in a class box which goes wherever the class does. Another has 'spacer stations' around the school.

Older children at secondary school are better able to use different inhalers, but, teenagers being teenagers, tend not to have their inhalers on them when they are needed! We recommend that they carry their own but that there should be a back-up in the medical room, in case. We don't believe that *preventer* medication should be kept in schools, because if it was administered by an untrained person when a child had an asthma attack it wouldn't work – that isn't what it's for.

If I was to give one piece of advice it would be that parents should make sure their child's medication was suitable for their age and understanding, ideally after seeing someone with specialist knowledge of asthma care. Asthma medication is simple and effective when you know how to use it! Parents should also be sure their child's school has an asthma policy in place and working. Increasingly, in schools this seems to be the case.

Teachers are sometimes worried about the possibility of theft or misuse of inhalers but in my experience that just hasn't been a problem.

We also run junior asthma clubs in some schools.

According to the asthma nurses we spoke to, schools have made huge efforts in the last ten years or so to include children with asthma in a normal school environment. As long as your child's asthma is well controlled with medication (and he remembers to take it!) and everyone at school knows about his asthma there's no reason why he shouldn't take a full part in ordinary school life.

7

'Will He Grow Out of It?'

One of the most frequently asked questions when a child has been diagnosed asthmatic is 'Will he grow out of it?' Unfortunately, there is no simple answer. More children are receiving treatment for asthma than adults – between 10 and 20 per cent of children and between 5 and 10 per cent of adults, according to the British Lung Foundation. There have been some long-term studies, beginning as long ago as the 1950s and 1960s, tracking people over the years and finding out more about the 'natural history' of asthma. They have shown that

- as many as 42 per cent of people in the UK have experienced some sort of wheezy illness by the time they reach their mid-thirties;
- there is a spectrum of asthma and wheezy illness, ranging from the very mild – which tends to disappear as children grow – to the very severe, which tends to persist into adult life;
- very severe childhood asthma which persists into adulthood tends to be associated with poor lung function in later life.

Because it's hard to diagnose asthma accurately in very young children, it's often difficult for your doctor to advise you about what will happen as your child grows up. Some studies suggest that as many as a third to a half of all young children have at least one 'wheezy' episode. However, many of these are caused by viral infections like bronchiolitis rather than by classic allergic asthma, which affects perhaps one in seven children over 5 years old.

Some children have lots of wheezy episodes in early childhood and later go on to show symptoms of classic, allergic asthma. Boys tend to be affected more commonly than girls, and babies born prematurely seem particularly at risk. Others, sometimes known as 'transient early wheezers', have wheezing episodes which are often associated with colds which they grow out of by the time they are in primary school.

Sometimes, asthma seems to 'disappear' as children grow into their teens only to resurface again when they are adults. Girls seem to catch up with boys at puberty and by the age of 18 there are slightly more female asthmatics than male. Put another way, it seems that boys are more likely than girls to 'grow out of it' – although, as we've said, more boys than girls have asthma to begin with. Babies and young children whose wheezing is associated with bronchiolitis and other viral infections, rather than allergic asthma, seem to have perfectly healthy lungs by the time they are in early middle age. Babies whose mothers smoked during pregnancy, and children growing up in homes where the adults smoke, are at higher risk of asthma, but according to the British Thoracic Society there is 'no identifiable association' between parental smoking and asthma in later life.

Clearly, there's a lot about asthma that we still don't know. It is also not unknown for people to develop asthma for the first time in their fifties. There is also the possibility that adults with a tendency to asthma and other allergic diseases will develop it after exposure to work-related pollutants.

Children whose asthma is severe and persistent, who have frequent attacks, and whose condition doesn't respond well to standard treatments with steroids and bronchodilators, seem to have poorer prospects as they grow up. Their lung function tends to deteriorate and persistent asthma, starting in childhood and persisting into adulthood, is sometimes associated with progressive damage to the airways. This is another reason why it's so important that childhood asthma is diagnosed and treated at as early a point as possible. Treatment isn't a once-and-for-all event. Whether your child's condition seems to be less troublesome, or more troublesome, as time passes, it will need to be carefully monitored by your GP, asthma nurse or specialist, so that the right levels of both preventer and reliever medication can be prescribed throughout childhood and into adult life.

No simple answer

There have been scientific studies of asthmatic children, monitoring them over the years to find out what happens to their asthma and general lung health in adult life. Generally speaking, whether a child goes on having asthma attacks in adult life seems to depend on the severity of the childhood illness, as well as personal and family history, although there are exceptions.

'Predictions for the future of asthmatic children are never easy,' says Dr Warren Lenny, Consultant Respiratory Paediatrician at the University Hospital of North Staffordshire.

It is a confusing picture, not least because it is still quite difficult to diagnose allergic asthma in young children. In the 1960s, doctors were talking about 'wheezy bronchitis' and prescribing antibiotics. Then in the 1970s it was thought that so-called 'wheezy bronchitis' was the mild end of the asthma spectrum and every wheeze was treated with asthma therapy. But not everything that wheezes is classic allergic asthma. Some children only wheeze when they are suffering from a cold virus. These children, if they are otherwise well and don't suffer from a persistent cough or an obvious allergy to pollen, animal dander or house-dust mite, are likely to lose their symptoms as they grow older. On the other hand a child who wheezes after exercise or reacts to allergens like house-dust mite may find his symptoms continue into adulthood.

It is complicated by the fact that childhood asthma symptoms tend to be intermittent. In one long-term follow-up study, 50 per cent of the children who had had asthma symptoms in early childhood were symptom-free by the time they were 7. But when they were looked at again at 11 and at 23, some had started wheezing again. Asthma can be very unpredictable.

Researchers in Australia found that 70 per cent of children whose asthma was very severe continued to have symptoms in adult life, compared to only about 20 per cent of children whose symptoms were mild. Family history plays a part too – in atopic families where other allergic conditions were present, asthma symptoms tended to continue.

Of course, as people get older other factors come into the equation, for instance smoking, or working in a dusty or smoky atmosphere. There are as many 20-year-old asthmatics who smoke as there are non-asthmatics. A study in my local area of Stoke and Wolverhampton found that between 17 and 30 per cent of 12–13-year-olds were smokers, which is worrying. As far as general lung health is concerned, a long-term study at Aberdeen University, looking at children from the mid-1970s onwards, found that those who had suffered from viral-induced wheeze had few lung symptoms by the age of 25, although those who had suffered from allergic asthma did. It's estimated that 60 per cent of Britain's adult population in 2012 will have suffered from childhood asthma symptoms at some point.

There is no simple answer to the 'will he grow out of it?' question, but what does seem likely is that children whose symptoms are mild, or only brought on by colds and other viral infections, have a better chance of becoming symptom-free in later life than those with severe allergic symptoms.

Symptoms can vary over time

Patricia's son David, who has asthma and anaphylaxis, finds that the severity of his symptoms has varied over time.

'When he was very small he would begin breathing very rapidly and go blue around the mouth,' Patricia remembers.

We used to rush him to hospital where a nebulizer was used to get the drugs into him. He had frequent attacks like that until he was prescribed preventer medication. I worried a bit about the side-effects of the steroids but they didn't seem to be a problem and his attacks of asthma were much reduced. Over time, we learned to manage the asthma much better. David's symptoms were always much worse in winter than summer so we adjusted his medication accordingly.

Now, he has been pretty much symptom-free for two years. He does try to look after himself when he has a cold and if he is ever exposed to his 'triggers' the effects are much less dramatic than they used to be. The longer we go on, the better controlled his asthma is. He is able to take part in all the usual activities including hockey and cross-country at school. His lungs seem to have become stronger and his airways less hyper-reactive.

Helping teenagers to manage their asthma

Asthma nurse Liz Biggart says that it can sometimes be a problem helping teenagers to manage their asthma, especially if their symptoms are relatively mild.

Teenagers are interested in becoming independent and this is not always matched by their understanding about how to control their asthma. With all the physical and social changes in puberty, the fact that a teenager has asthma can sometimes be resented, or even ignored. Boys, in particular, may deny they have a problem or decide to 'tough it out' by refusing to carry or use their medication, even when they need it. Some are just not self-disciplined enough to take regular medication, and of course parents are not in control as they were when the child was younger. This can cause a lot of worry.

Liz advises gently suggesting to young people that they listen to their body so that they can understand what's happening and can minimize any problems. For instance, teens who are keen on sport can be reminded that five minutes' preventer medication, morning and evening, will get their asthma under control and enable them to take part in exactly the same activities as their friends. This could also be the time to remind them that sporting heroes like Paula Radcliffe or Manchester United soccer star Paul Scholes are both asthmatics.

Liz comments:

All teenagers think they are immortal, and they want to be able to go out to clubs and bars and even smoke if their friends do. Teenagers don't appreciate lectures, but they like to make their own decisions from an informed perspective. Smoking, of course, is extremely damaging, and especially so for those with asthma.

If you are concerned about your teenagers smoking – and, sadly, there is quite a lot of evidence that teenage girls, especially, are still smoking because it's seen as 'cool' and helps to keep them slim – telling them about the health risks doesn't always work, even if they are asthmatic. You might have more success if you remind them how much of their money is going up in smoke. Action on Smoking and Health (address on p. 80) estimate that a 20-a-day smoker who gives up will save between £1,600 and £1,700 in a year. That's enough to pay for a holiday *and* a sound system, with something left over for clothes . . .

And talking of clothes, you could also appeal to their vanity. Who was it said that snogging a smoker was like licking an ash-tray?

Of course, not all teenage asthmatics are so careless of their health. Some are quite health-conscious anyway. If they are used to controlling their own medication and having a say in their own 'asthma management plan', or if they have been frightened into taking care by a bad asthma attack, they may be more willing to co-operate. Some of the National Asthma Campaign's helpful and easy-to-understand leaflets (details on p. 78) could give them all the information they need to help them make the right decisions.

There have been some imaginative schemes to encourage teen-agers to remember their asthma medication, including a trial in Scotland involving a mobile text messaging service. With so many youngsters apparently welded to their mobiles, this could easily be adapted by parents wanting to remind their kids to use their medication. In the Scottish scheme, 32 young people with asthma from the Tayside area were recruited through the local radio station and sent regular text messages by a 'virtual friend with asthma' called Max. Max used contemporary text jargon and the teenagers involved in the project participated enthusiastically. Many sent text messages back to Max letting him know that they had remembered to take their medication and reporting that they were less likely to forget when Max was there to remind them.

Asthma and career choice

Young people with asthma will also need to take their condition into account when they are starting to think about career choices. Obviously, any job which would involve working somewhere with poor air quality, somewhere dusty or somewhere they would be exposed to fumes or excessive pollen, would be likely to trigger an asthma attack and should be avoided. Similarly, youngsters who know that animal dander makes them wheeze have to say no to careers caring for animals. There's also a question-mark over careers in the emergency services or Armed Forces. A history of severe asthma would probably rule these careers out, although mild childhood asthma which has not persisted might not do so. The police, for instance, say that each case is assessed individually, and the Army point out that soldiers may be exposed to gases, so any treatment for asthma in the preceding four years should be stated on any application form. Firefighters and ambulance paramedics are often exposed to smoke and other pollutants, making these careers inappropriate for asthma sufferers. Fortunately, non-smoking offices are now becoming the norm as the effects of 'passive smoking' on everyone, not just those with breathing difficulties, become better known.

Letting go

It isn't easy for any parent, particularly the parent of a child with asthma, to 'let go' and allow teenagers more freedom, including the freedom to make mistakes! If your child is planning to go away to university all you can do is remind him to be aware of his asthma triggers and always carry his medication. Once he has college accommodation arranged, make sure his flatmates, friends and the staff are aware that he has asthma. It's also important that he registers as soon as possible with a GP who should be aware of his condition.

It's even more important that your student son or daughter's friends and the college staff know if he or she also suffers from other allergies or anaphylaxis.

'We have sent information about severe allergic reactions to colleges and universities so that they are aware of the problem, but our members report that some are more helpful than others,' says a spokeswoman for the Anaphylaxis Campaign. Student members of the campaign recommend telling all your friends about the risk of anaphylaxis and making sure they know what to do if you have a severe reaction. Some catering managers in catered halls are very sympathetic to those who have to have special diets, or students might prefer to self-cater.

The Campaign has just produced a booklet called *Letting Go – Teaching an Allergic Child Responsibility* which is full of helpful advice for parents of older children and adolescents. Parents of any child with a chronic health condition are caught between the natural urge to protect, and knowing that their child has to learn to be independent and eventually manage the condition alone. Although this booklet is aimed at the parents of children with anaphylaxis, there are useful tips for parents of asthmatics too – on staying calm, teaching children self-esteem so that they can cope with peer pressure and say 'No' when necessary, and encouraging youngsters to take responsibility for their own health and medication. The booklet is available from the Anaphylaxis Campaign (address on p. 79).

8

Complementary Medicine

Most cases of childhood asthma respond well to conventional medicine. Normally, a combination of preventer medication and relievers to be used when necessary will be all your child needs to keep her asthma under control. Nor is there any indication that current treatments have unwanted or dangerous side-effects.

So why turn to complementary therapies? There is little scientific evidence that they work. Very few of the large-scale, double-blind, placebo-controlled clinical trials which conventional medicines have to go through before they are put on the market have ever been undertaken for complementary therapies. Any trials which have taken place are often inconclusive. Some doctors are dismissive, like Joe Neary of the Royal College of General Practitioners.

> We have evidence on our side. There is no evidence that complementary therapies help children with asthma. Some have claimed that homoeopathy is an effective treatment, but when it was tested, any benefits were not statistically significant. Any responsible complementary therapist will tell you to carry on using the steroids and bronchodilators, even if you use complementary medicine too.

Not all experts are quite so dismissive. The National Asthma Campaign has a factsheet on complementary therapies, and reports that membership surveys suggest that some people find them helpful. They recommend that anyone thinking of trying any kind of complementary treatment should discuss it with their doctor first. It's also important to make sure that the therapist you work with is a member of the appropriate professional organization (see pp. 81–2) and is properly trained and qualified. The NAC actively encourages research into complementary treatments, as it's difficult to recommend any kind of treatment unless it has been properly studied, evaluated and written up in reputable medical journals. The World Health Organization's Global Strategy for Asthma also recognizes the need for more research before recommendations can be made.

Acupuncture

The NAC reports that acupuncture, for example, can sometimes have short-term beneficial effects on asthma, though it is said to be less effective in those whose asthma is triggered by exercise. Again, more research is needed.

Laura has found that both acupuncture and acupressure (which doesn't use needles) have helped her severely asthmatic and allergic son and reduced the levels of bronchodilator drugs he needs to take.

The NAC said that acupuncture might work and my GP, who is severely asthmatic herself, tried it. She was so impressed that she invited an acupuncturist to join the GP practice!

At first it was difficult to find an acupuncturist with experience of working with children. My son was 8, and acupressure was recommended for him. As he got older, he started having acupuncture. After the sessions, which lasted about an hour, he would say that he felt as though an elastic band had been removed from his chest. I could see his chest walls lift, his shoulders drop, and his breathing become more relaxed.

In winter he has a session about once every two months and in summer or when the pollen count is especially high, it could be as often as once a week.

Homoeopathy

There is some debate among scientists at the moment about the possible value of homoeopathy as a treatment for asthma. Dr Adrian White, Senior Lecturer in Complementary Medicine at the Peninsula Medical School in Exeter, recently conducted a double-blind, placebo-controlled trial of homoeopathic remedies, where 96 children with moderate asthma were prescribed either a homoeopathic remedy or a placebo. It was found that there were no significant changes in symptoms, use of medication or quality of life in the group using the remedy – in other words, homoeopathy had no effect on the children's asthma.

Diet

Some complementary therapists advocate a change of diet as a way of reducing asthma symptoms, but according to the NAC the benefits of this are unclear. Children who have proven allergies to certain foods – most commonly dairy products, wheat or nuts – should, of course, avoid coming into contact with them, but otherwise there's no real evidence that changing your child's diet will help.

Government guidelines state that if you have asthma or other allergic disease in the family, it's best for mums-to-be to avoid eating peanuts or peanut products during pregnancy and while breast-feeding. Otherwise, there's no evidence that changing your diet during pregnancy will help to prevent your baby from developing childhood asthma.

Herbal medicines

Herbal medicines have a very long history both in Britain and abroad. Many of the drugs we take for granted today have their origins in herbal preparations. Sometimes herbal treatments are recommended for asthma but, again, few have been put through rigorous scientific tests.

Herbal remedies, like conventional medicines, can have side-effects, can react with other medication (including asthma medication) and can be poisonous. This means it is essential to tell your doctor what you are thinking of giving your child, and also to make sure any herbal practitioner you consult is a member of the National Institute of Medical Herbalists.

Catherine Acott is a medical herbalist whose own 7-year-old daughter has asthma. She also treats asthmatic children with herbal remedies.

The first thing I tell parents is not to throw away the inhalers, although, if I am doing my job properly, the child's need for Ventolin and Becotide should drop away. Today's asthma clinics are generally good at monitoring children and will recommend a reduction in the use of steroid treatments as the child's condition improves.

When a child is brought to me I try to establish whether the wheezing is post-viral – in which case I would prescribe herbs like echinacea to strengthen the immune system – or whether it is caused by an allergy. Some children do improve if they avoid cow's milk products, but it does vary. Chocolate makes my daughter wheeze and cough. Every child is different.

I would look at the family history, asking the same questions as a GP. A prescription may include five to seven different herbs, usually in the form of a tincture which can be added to something like apple juice, as most children prefer cold to hot drinks.

The skill of herbalism lies in combining herbs to suit a particular child. Herbs like chamomile, plantain and eyebright can be used to mediate an allergic reaction. Chamomile also has an anti-inflammatory action, as does liquorice. For an irritating cough I might prescribe marsh mallow, and hyssop or plantain, again, for excess mucus.

It is important not to take chances with a condition which can be dangerous. I find that young patients are very good at avoiding their 'triggers' once they know what they are and will happily tell other people what they can't eat. My daughter and I have found other treats to replace chocolate!

Pycnogenol

One nutritional supplement which is said to be effective in improving the airway function of asthmatics is an extract of French pine bark called Pycnogenol. Many of the nutrients found in Pycnogenol are bioflavonoids, which are anti-oxidant compounds found in many plants. A small scientific study in the USA found that treatment with Pycnogenol improved adult patients' ability to exhale (breathe out) and also reduced the levels of leukotrienes in the blood. Leukotrienes are the 'chemical messengers' which are released in the body by some cell types and react on others, amplifying the inflammation and irritation of the airways. Most recently, Dr Benjamin Lau at Loma Linda University in California has been studying Pycnogenol as a treatment for children. The research project is not yet completed but Dr Lau says that in his own practice he finds it helpful.

I have helped many children to keep their asthma under control with the use of complementary therapies, including Pycnogenol. One of the things we do is find out what triggers asthma attacks. In the USA, many children are allergic to dairy products and refined sugars. By removing these two items we eliminate many of their complaints. Cow's milk is the most mucus-forming substance that causes bronchospasm. Refined sugars lower one's resistance to fight infections. In our practice, we find that Pycnogenol works like corticosteroids, but without any side-effects.

Yoga and Buteyko

Among the most interesting complementary therapies for asthma are those which involve special breathing exercises, like yoga and Buteyko, both of which are suitable for children and teenagers.

Again, there don't seem to be many scientific studies on this but both techniques can relieve stress, which can sometimes be an asthma trigger.

Robin Monroe is Director of the Yoga Biomedical Trust, a registered charity (contact details on p. 82). He says that yoga has great potential as a treatment for asthma.

I was an asthmatic child myself and was cured in my thirties by taking up yoga. With young children, much will depend on the parents' level of involvement and understanding. Relaxation plays a big part and there are specific exercises children can be taught from the age of about 6 or 7. They can begin to learn breathing with movement, as well as postures which will help them to open up their chests and breathe out fully. Children with asthma are often very tense around their chests and shoulders and tend to panic and tense up even more when they have an asthma attack.

The kinds of yoga which incorporate breathing techniques are most valuable, rather than those which just teach postures. Asthma is associated with hyperventilation and yoga is about re-training the breathing, tuning into each breath and slowing it down. When a person is tense their breath is forced. When they relax, the body naturally comes back to its own proper rhythm. We teach a sequence of breathing exercises which can be used during asthma attacks. Postures also have a role to play. A posture like the Cobra involves extending the back and opening up the shoulders, and this can help asthmatics. Even quite small children can be taught yoga via games and play and often enjoy the postures and the exercises.

We would never recommend giving up medication but this often happens naturally when the child's symptoms improve. Children find they don't need to use their inhalers so often and GPs have to check to see whether they still need preventer medication.

Buteyko is a special breathing technique developed by a Russian professor more than fifty years ago. It is said to work by altering the balance of oxygen and carbon dioxide in the air which is breathed out. Those who believe in the technique say that people with asthma 'over-breathe' or hyperventilate when there is no need to do so and that this results in irritation, inflammation and constriction of the airways.

'We aren't anti-drugs,' says Buteyko spokesman Kim Upton.

But we do enable people with asthma to use their medication less and less. I was asthmatic myself from the age of 10 and found that as time went on I was having to use more and more of my medication. I know now that the drugs I was taking were actually aggravating my problem by upsetting my breathing patterns. Professor Buteyko believed that the function of our respiratory system was not just to push air in and out, but also to maintain the right ratio of oxygen to carbon dioxide. He observed that asthmatics had low carbon dioxide levels, and that was why their muscles went into spasm. Carbon dioxide relaxes the muscles of the airways.

Kim says that the method is especially suitable for children as it doesn't take them so long to un-learn their faulty breathing habits.

'We find that children are able to reduce their medication very quickly,' he comments. 'I have seen children who had no energy, couldn't join in sports and games and were using nebulizers come back after a week with colour in their cheeks and looking completely different!'

Fiona's 13-year-old daughter Jordan was a 'chesty' baby who was diagnosed with asthma when she was 4. The family lived in South Africa for a time where the outdoor life seemed to suit Jordan, but on their return to England she had continual severe colds accompanied by asthma attacks.

In the end she was taking steroids in the morning and evening plus a Ventolin inhaler when she needed it during the daytime, but the asthma was still not really controlled. She was on courses of steroid tablets for three or five days at a time sometimes, too. In the autumn of 2002 I took her for a check-up at our local hospital who wanted to hospitalize her because her medication didn't seem to be working.

However, I had just booked up for a Buteyko course which I had read about and wanted to try, rather than relying on even more doses of steroids. It was absolutely brilliant. The exercises are all about controlled breathing, or under-breathing. I had been telling her to take deep breaths, which was completely the wrong advice! Jordan was taught to hold her breath and walk up and down the room. At first she could only do 20 paces, now she is up to 80 or 90. We were also told about diet and lifestyle changes but quite honestly we haven't done anything special. I just watch out for Jordan getting wheezy and advise her not to eat too much chocolate or dairy products. We never ate many convenience foods anyway.

Jordan does her breathing exercises morning and evening, and is now down to using just the one steroid inhaler as a preventer. She has had maybe five puffs of Ventolin since she went on the Buteyko course and we are hoping that if she improves any more she will be able to give up medication altogether. My GP and hospital doctors were sceptical, so I plan to take Jordan in to see them and show them the improvement in her health!

A scientific research study in Australia indicated that Buteyko could indeed help with asthma symptoms and the NAC funded further research into the method as an addition to more conventional treatment. They found that it did help to reduce symptoms in some people, who then needed to use their reliever inhalers less frequently, but didn't improve the underlying condition. They say that Buteyko does appear to help asthmatics feel more in control and 'may be worth trying'.

The Hale Clinic

The Hale Clinic in London is one of the country's best-known centres for complementary medicine. Dr George Georgiou, a therapist there, is also Director of the Natural Therapy Centre at Larnaca in Cyprus. He has wide experience of working with children with asthma.

'Each child has its own biochemical and physiological individuality and we need to discover what these are and address them accordingly,' he says.

The first question I ask is always, 'Why does this child have asthma and related symptoms?' Many factors could be responsible for putting such a burden on a child's immune system. Then the detective work begins.

Among the factors involved could be: stored toxins from food or drugs; vaccination stress; geopathic stress; food intolerance (caused by items such as iced water, ice cream, fruits, juices, wheat, chocolate, dairy products and nuts); anti-oxidant deficiency; tooth and scar foci, in older children; or candidiasis caused by the over-use of antibiotics.

Once he has identified the cause of the problem, Dr Georgiou treats the patient with an individually tailor-made programme which may incorporate homoeopathic remedies, herbal medicines, nutritional supplements, elimination diets and other elements which have been specifically tested to determine whether they are suitable for that particular child.

I find that a shotgun technique using natural remedies, just to suppress symptoms, is not the most effective way of treating the condition. Using a tailor-made programme, however, I find that in two or three months the symptoms of asthma begin to disappear as the child's body finds the strength to begin repairing itself. Nature is doing the healing. Many children find they can stop taking steroids and using nebulizers and so on within two or three months, if they follow a programme that is individually devised for them.

Osteopathy

Osteopathy, a system of healing based on the manipulation of bones, is probably more associated with the treatment of bad backs than asthma. However, the British College of Osteopathic Medicine (contact details on p. 81) actually runs a free children's clinic. Like yoga and Buteyko, above, treatment is partly based on teaching better breathing techniques. According to Lawrence Kirk, Dean of Clinical Studies (who suffered from childhood asthma himself), therapists take a three-pronged approach. Treatment consists of a combination of the physical, biochemical/nutritional and emotional.

Children with asthma often show postural changes. They use their muscles and joints differently from other children, in trying to get more air into their lungs during asthma attacks. Normal, healthy breathing uses the diaphragm. Asthmatics tend to panic and use all their muscles, which can impact on their heads, necks, chests and spines and the attached muscles. In the long term, these muscles can become overtaxed and strained, sometimes leading to permanent damage and postural changes.

What we try to do is teach children to use their diaphragms effectively when they breathe. Asthmatics frequently don't realize, but their problem is often breathing *out* effectively, rather than trying to breathe *in*.

Children sometimes find it hard to co-ordinate their breathing so we have devised fun exercises to help them to breathe more effectively. Exercises might involve rhythmic panting to try to encourage air to come out, especially during wheezy episodes. Then there is singing – singing a long note also encourages exhalation. Children are shown how to make animal-type noises so that they can actually feel their diaphragm working as it should.

As well as the breathing exercises, the College encourages a holistic approach to asthma care which is designed to complement, not replace, conventional medication. Advice on nutrition may be given. A diet rich in fruit and vegetables is said to benefit lung function. Fish oils – found in fish like salmon and tuna – are recommended. Additives like tartrazine (E102) are said to be a source of irritation in some susceptible people. Parents of asthmatic children are advised to try and cut down on possible allergens in the home. Emotional and psychological issues are also confronted. Lawrence Kirk says that he can remember feeling guilty, as an asthmatic child, for keeping his father awake at night by coughing!

As he points out:

Stress can impact on the illness, and the more information parents and children have, the easier it is to maintain a calm atmosphere at home. Parents also need to guard against being over-protective, although this is sometimes difficult. For instance, many asthmatics do benefit from exercise. I belong to a rugby club where I would say 15 or 20 per cent of the younger players use inhalers before a match but they still enjoy playing rugby. Sport, especially swimming, promotes general well-being and improves lung function.

A word of warning

The NAC point out that some complementary products can actually be dangerous for people with asthma. Among them are Royal Jelly and Propolis, products produced by bees and sold as health supplements. Apparently, some people with asthma and similar allergic conditions have suffered from extremely severe reactions to these products, and in Australia, Royal Jelly products now carry a health warning stating that they should not be taken by people with asthma or allergies. Although Propolis has not been shown to have such severe side-effects, caution is advised because it is also a bee product.

The British Thoracic Society, in its most recent guidelines on asthma management, also came to the conclusion that a lot more research was needed before any form of complementary therapy could be recommended. Even where trials had taken place, either the methodology was suspect or the results were inconclusive.

For instance, they quoted 17 trials of herbal or Chinese medicine, where nine reported an improvement in lung function, but said that it wasn't clear whether these findings could apply to Britain. Another single trial found that acupuncture had a beneficial effect on asthma, but was less effective than current drugs. Air ionizers, which are often advertised as of benefit to asthma sufferers, have not been scientifically proved to work. Hypnosis, the report says 'may be effective', but more research is required. The BTS was equally cautious about recommending breathing exercises, like those pre-scribed in yoga or Buteyko, and by some physiotherapists, which some people with asthma apparently find helpful.

Changes in diet are also sometimes suggested by 'alternative' practitioners but, again, the results of the few random clinical trials are inconclusive. One study suggested that magnesium supplements might help to prevent wheeze, although antioxidant supplements such as Vitamin C and selenium have not been proved to work. Omega-3 fish oils have been prescribed as a way of reducing the inflammation associated with asthma but, again, there is little evidence that they help. Both adults and children who are very overweight do find asthma management easier when they lose those excess kilos, however.

It's important to remember that none of the trials mentioned in the British Thoracic Society report were conducted on children – which means that there's even less evidence for the effectiveness of complementary therapies on children with asthma.

However, as anyone who has used complementary therapies knows, the fact that they haven't been scientifically proved to work doesn't mean that they don't! If you normally use herbal or homoeopathic medicines for minor ailments, and you are working with a qualified medical herbalist or homoeopathic doctor you trust, you could ask them if there's anything they would recommend for your child that can be used *alongside* more conventional medication.

9

What about the Future?

It doesn't look as though a cure for asthma is in sight. Even though the condition is estimated to cost the National Health Service about £670 million in drug treatments, GP consultations and hospital visits, it's a bit of a poor relation when research funds are being handed out. According to the British Lung Foundation, the charities which fund all forms of lung research in Britain are able to spend just £6 million on research every year – less than a third of what a political party can spend on a General Election campaign.

However, there is positive news. At the moment, doctors treating asthmatic children say that their goal is to get the child's asthma under control so that she can live a normal life. More and better drugs, and better ways of delivering medication, are part of that. There is also considerable research taking place into *why* so many of today's children are developing asthma. Prevention, after all, is better than cure.

Prevention – a priority for research

Respiratory epidemiologist Dr Seif Shaheen of King's College in London feels that preventing asthma occurring in the first place is one of the most worthwhile areas for research.

We may have some answers within the next five years. At the moment researchers are looking into factors in pregnancy because it is thought that the causes of asthma might start very early in life – before a baby is even born. We already know that asthma is more common in low-birthweight babies, premature babies, and the babies of mothers who smoke. We are also looking at whether maternal diet plays a part, at the influence of antioxidant vitamins and fatty acids. We may have more information in a couple of years. After that clinical trials will have to be set up, and after that we may be in a position to advise mums-to-be on a better diet. Researchers have already looked at the influence of items like apples, fruit and vegetables generally, and the mineral selenium. A diet rich in fruit and vegetables seems to be a good idea for all sorts of reasons and we will know more as research progresses.

Obesity is another area that is being looked at. Fatter children do have more asthma, and obesity among the general public is increasing although, as yet, we have no evidence that one is responsible for the other. In the past two or three years there have been studies linking overweight with asthma and it is helpful if people with asthma lose weight.

It has also been suggested that there might be a link between the use of paracetamol and the increase in childhood asthma, although any research on this is at a very early stage. This may be because in the mid-1980s paracetamol began to replace aspirin as the treatment for childhood fevers, and this coincided with the increase in the numbers of children diagnosed with asthma. However, there is no proof yet of a causal link. We know that mothers who use paracetamol during pregnancy are more likely to have children who wheeze, so it's possible that some children are susceptible, but it is too early to be sure whether this is the case.

The general public feels intuitively that pollution probably plays a part in the increase in the number of cases, but it's a complex subject. Pollution doesn't cause asthma, though it can act as a trigger in some individuals. Our air has got cleaner in the last twenty years with the advent of lead-free petrol and so on, but the type of pollution in the atmosphere has changed. And there are some things that we just can't explain, like why there should be more asthma on the Isle of Skye, with its clean air, than there is on the Scottish mainland.

There is also the possibility of a vaccine, similar in type to the BCG vaccine which is used against tuberculosis.

The National Asthma Campaign agrees that 'primary prevention' – stopping children from developing asthma – is a priority area for research, and has a team of scientists working on this.

'We know there is a genetic element, in that children whose parents have asthma are more likely to have it too. We also know that environmental factors play a part,' says their spokesman.

What we don't yet know is exactly which environmental factors, or how they interact with each other, but in the next couple of years we could have some answers. At the moment we are looking at large groups of children who have been 'tracked' from birth to the early teens, and trying to work out why some have developed asthma while others are asthma-free.

Professor Peter Jeffrey, a lung pathologist at London's Royal

Brompton Hospital, is working on research with Finnish colleagues which is aimed at predicting which 'wheezy' babies later go on to develop asthma and why. They are looking at the membrane that supports the cells lining babies' airways. The idea is to find out whether the thickening which is characteristic of asthma is already present in very young babies, or is caused by chronic inflammation. This is a long-term research project lasting at least seven years but should help doctors to detect asthma earlier in children's lives.

Another NAC research project at the University of Aberdeen is looking at the influence of maternal diet on children's asthma. Dr Graham Devereux and his team are studying 2,000 children as a follow-up to earlier research which found that children whose mothers had a high Vitamin E intake during pregnancy were less sensitive to allergens. The team is now looking at the children's eating habits, lung function and any allergies they have. In future, it may be possible to give mums-to-be specific dietary advice aimed at asthma avoidance.

Developing vaccines

Other scientists are working on the development of vaccines against asthma and other allergic conditions. Dr Mark Larche is a Senior Research Fellow for the NAC and works at the National Heart and Lung Institute at Imperial College in London. He is working on what is known as 'desensitizing immunotherapy' which involves injecting susceptible subjects with progressively larger doses of the substances they're allergic to, in order to desensitize them.

He is hoping that a vaccine against cat allergy may be licensed by 2006 or 2007. Trials have already been carried out using a first prototype, which has shown that allergic responses in people can be regulated. Larger trials are now beginning. At the same time the research team is working on similar vaccines for house-dust mites and pollen.

It was recently reported that a Swedish company was working on a vaccine which would work against all kinds of allergy, including hay-fever and pet allergy. This is said to work by stimulating the immune system to destroy its own IgE antibody so that the allergic response does not occur. Professor Lars Hellman of Uppsala University said that if forthcoming clinical trials succeed it will be a major scientific breakthrough, but that the vaccine was still some years in the future.

New treatments

As far as new treatments are concerned, inhaled steroids have been the front-line treatment for asthma for the last twenty years, and they are very good at dealing with inflamed airways. In the last few years new drugs have come on to the market called Leukotriene Receptor Antagonists or LRTAs, which also have the effect of damping down inflammation of the airways. They can be used in conjunction with steroids, or as another step in the treatment of asthma, and they work for some people. Another drug called an anti-IgE monoclonal antibody, which targets the allergic component of asthma, has been used in the USA but isn't yet licensed in this country.

Better management

The NAC is also keen to help patients, including children, manage their own treatment better. Like diabetics, those who have asthma need to keep taking medication – in their case, steroids – when they may be feeling perfectly well. It is always tempting to skip a dose, or doses, because you feel you don't need them. It's often difficult to persuade older children and teenagers that they need their medication without sounding like 'fussy old Mum'. The more young people understand about asthma and the better informed they are, the more likely it is that they will go on taking their preventer medication and so avoid flare-ups.

Nurses are playing an increasing part in asthma management. Some are running GP and hospital asthma clinics, while others are going out into the community to advise schools on the most appropriate way to care for children with asthma. Dr Warren Lenny, Consultant Respiratory Paediatrician at the University Hospital of North Staffordshire, says that in the future most asthma patients will be looked after by teams of nurses, including at least one nurse who is a specialist in childhood asthma.

'In our hospital we are building up a patient database and making sure that all cases get a follow-up consultation with the nursing team within a week,' he says. 'GP asthma clinics also play a part and so far we have found this system to be popular with the parents of children with asthma.'

Other research projects

The British Lung Foundation has funded almost 100 asthma research projects. Five years ago, scientists they support identified an antibody in the blood of asthmatics which could lead to the development of a vaccine. They have also funded a research project in Nottingham looking at exactly how the house-dust mite allergen causes an allergic reaction. This kind of research is much needed, because at the moment families with an asthmatic child are often advised to avoid allergens, sometimes by making expensive lifestyle changes like replacing carpets with wooden floors, without proper proof that these allergen-avoidance strategies actually work.

The BLF also say that the treatment of very young children – under 2 years old – is, at present, unsatisfactory as they don't respond very well to the current range of treatments.

Researchers have found that asthma in early childhood is not a single disease but a combination of disorders with similar symptoms like coughing and wheezing – some caused by allergic asthma, others by viral infections – for which different treatments may be appropriate.

Researchers funded by the BLF discovered that babies can recognize the allergens their mothers are exposed to by the twenty-second week of pregnancy.

10
Further Help

Asthma can't yet be cured but it can be managed, and there are lots of people out there who can help you and your child to manage it. It has been found that asthma patients do better if they feel they are in control, and the more information you have about the condition, the more in control you feel. In addition to your GP, asthma nurse, hospital specialist and/or physio, here are some of the people who can help you.

The National Asthma Campaign
Providence House
Providence Place
London N1 0NT

Helpline: 0845 701 0203 (9 a.m.–5 p.m., Mon.–Fri.)
Website: www.asthma.org.uk

The National Asthma Campaign Scotland
2a North Charlotte Street
Edinburgh EH2 4HR

Tel: 0131 226 2544
Website: www.asthma.org.uk

The NAC campaigns for more resources and better treatment for asthma patients, both adults and children, and wants the government and the NHS to make asthma a priority. It funds research projects into the causes of and treatments for asthma. It can provide a wealth of helpful literature on all aspects of the condition, including the 'Be in Control' material which incorporates your child's own individual asthma plan. It also has special Schools Packs which heads and teachers can obtain to help them integrate children with asthma into all kinds of schools. The NAC was made Boots Charity of the Year in 2003.

To mark World Asthma Day in May 2003, the NAC produced its Asthma Charter for patients to take to their GP, to ensure they are receiving the recommended standards of care (see Appendix 2, p. 85).

The Anaphylaxis Campaign
P.O. Box 275
Farnborough
Hants GU14 6SX

Helpline: 01252 542029
Website www.anaphylaxis.org.uk

The Campaign offers information and guidance for those suffering from extreme and life-threatening allergies. It also campaigns for better awareness of the problem and for better food labelling.

Allergy UK
Deepdene House
30 Bellegrove Road
Welling
Kent DA16 3PY

Allergy helpline: 020 8303 8583 (9 a.m.–9 p.m. weekdays)
Chemical sensitivity helpline: 020 8303 8525 (9 a.m.–5 p.m. weekdays)
Website: www.allergyuk.org

Allergy UK has information on all forms of allergy, including common asthma 'triggers' and how to avoid them. Offers factsheets, leaflets, a magazine and lists of useful products like anti-allergy bed-linen and recommended vacuum cleaners.

British Lung Foundation
78 Hatton Garden
London EC1N 8LD

Tel: 020 7831 5831
Website: www.lunguk.org

The BLF works throughout the country to improve the prevention, diagnosis and treatment of all lung diseases, including asthma. It runs Breathe Easy clubs for people affected by breathing problems. It also has advice and information leaflets on topics like indoor and outdoor air pollution.

Cats Protection
17 Kings Road
Horsham
West Sussex RH13 5PN

Helpline: 01403 221919
Website: www.cats.org.uk

Cats Protection has a leaflet *Do You Have Asthma?* with hints on asthma management for cat-owners and those considering getting a cat.

The WellBeing/Sainsbury's Eating for Pregnancy Helpline on 0845 130 3646 can offer up-to-date advice on healthy eating for mums-to-be. It is open from 10 a.m. to 4 p.m., Monday to Friday.

Quitline
Helpline: 0800 00 22 00 (9 a.m.–9 p.m. every day)
Website: www.quit.org.uk

For help in giving up smoking.

Action on Smoking and Health
NHS smoking helpline: 0800 169 0 169 (7 a.m.–11 p.m. every day)
Website: www.ash.org.uk

For help in giving up smoking.

Consumers' Association Subscription Line 0800 252 100
Website: www.which.co.uk

The CA publishes magazines including *Which?* and *Health Which?* which carry news reports on health issues including asthma, and test products like anti-allergy bedding and vacuum cleaners.

The Healthy House
The Old Co-op
Lower Street
Ruscombe
Stroud
Glos GL6 6BU

Tel: 01453 752216
Website: www.healthy-house.co.uk

Mail-order company selling allergy-free products, including house-dust mite sprays, pet sprays and dust mite-proof bedding.

Medivac Healthcare
Freepost
LON 12778 NW11 6YR

Tel: 0845 130 6164

Mail-order company selling anti-allergy bed-linen plus 'Medivac' and 'Medivap' vacuum cleaners with special filters designed to remove allergens.

The Pre-School Learning Alliance
69 King's Cross Road
London WC1X 9LL

Tel: 020 7833 0991
Website: www.pre-school.org.uk

The Pre-School Learning Alliance can help nursery nurses, play-group leaders and so on work out how to manage asthma in young children, with the co-operation of parents.

National Childminding Association
8 Masons Hill
Bromley
Kent BR2 9EY

Tel: 0800 169 4486 (10 a.m.–4 p.m., Mon.–Fri.)
Website: www.ncma.org.uk

The National Childminding Association can offer help and advice to parents and childminders.

The Department for Education and Skills can send heads and teachers or interested parents a copy of their report and fact pack *Supporting Pupils with Medical Needs*. Call 0845 602 2260.

Complementary therapies

The British College of Osteopathic Medicine
Lief House
3 Sumpter Close
120–122 Finchley Road
London NW3 5HR

Tel: 020 7435 6464
Website: www.bcom.ac.uk

For information about osteopathy as a treatment for asthma.

Kim Upton
Buteyko Health
Flat 55, Waldemar Mansions
Waldemar Avenue
London SW6 5LX

Tel: 020 7736 7670
Website: www.buteykohealth.com

For information about Buteyko courses.

The Yoga Therapy Centre and Yoga Biomedical Trust
90–92 Pentonville Road
Islington
London N1 9HS

Tel: 020 7689 3040
Website: www.yogatherapy.org

For details of yoga courses.

British Wheel of Yoga
25 Jermyn Street
Sleaford
Lincs NG34 7RU

Tel: 01529 306851
Website: www.bwy.org.uk

For information about yoga courses all over the country.

The Hale Clinic
7 Park Crescent
London W1B 1PF

Tel: 0870 167 6667
Website: www.haleclinic.com

For a range of complementary therapies including treatments for asthma.

National Institute of Medical Herbalists
56 Longbrook Street
Exeter
Devon EX4 6AH

Tel: 01392 426022
Website: www.nimh.org.uk

Acupuncture Council
63 Jeddo Road
London W12 9HQ

Tel: 020 8735 0400
Website: www.acupuncture.org.uk

Appendix 1
Vital Facts to Remember about Asthma

1 It is caused by a combination of inherited and environmental factors and seems to have become much more common in recent years. As yet, no one knows why.
2 It is difficult to diagnose in very young children. Not all wheezy or 'chesty' babies have, or will develop, asthma.
3 As yet there is no cure, but the condition can be managed.
4 The aim of asthma treatment is to enable your child to live a normal life and do everything other children do. All but a small minority of asthmatics can achieve this.
5 Asthma management is about teamwork. You, your child, your GP, your asthma nurse and/or chest specialist should be working together to help your child. Nurseries, schools, wider family and friends all have their part to play.
6 Modern asthma treatments, in the form of inhaled drugs, are very effective at controlling asthma. If a particular treatment seems not to suit your child, ask if she can try another.
7 It's vital that you and your child understand how his medication works and how to use it. Don't be afraid to ask questions if there's something you don't understand.
8 The National Asthma Campaign is there to help with lots of information about every aspect of childhood asthma. They deserve your support.
9 It is not possible to predict whether or not your child will grow out of asthma.
10 It's vital that everyone who takes care of your child knows that he has asthma, knows where to find and how to use his medication, and knows what to do in an emergency.
11 Asthma is a condition that needs monitoring. Even if your child's asthma is well controlled, she will need to see your GP or an asthma nurse regularly.
12 Asthma affects different children differently. Learn to recognize the factors that trigger an asthma attack in your child.
13 Having said that, you can't keep an active youngster in a protective bubble. Effective medication, plus a reasonable level of allergen avoidance, should enable your whole family to live a normal life.

14 The single most effective thing which parents can do to help their asthmatic child is give up smoking.

15 A healthy, balanced diet with plenty of fresh fruit and vegetables, plus exercise (preceded by a puff or two from an inhaler if necessary) will assist your child's immune system to resist the bugs that can cause respiratory infections. It will also help your child to maintain a healthy weight.

16 Some people find complementary therapies which involve breathing exercises, like yoga and Buteyko, beneficial. However, no reputable complementary therapist should suggest you give up your child's asthma medication.

Appendix 2
The Asthma Charter

As a person with asthma, I have a right to:

1 high-quality treatment, care and information from asthma-trained health professionals who know about best practice and the latest evidence;
2 access a doctor or nurse who has had specific asthma training, at either my local GP practice or in my local area;
3 have my asthma quickly and accurately diagnosed, with referral to a respiratory specialist if necessary;
4 a full and open discussion with my nurse about the best asthma treatments for me, including side-effects, regardless of the cost of the treatment;
5 be shown how to use the devices needed to keep my asthma under control (e.g. inhalers and spacers);
6 discuss and agree my own personal asthma plan with my doctor or nurse, so that I can keep my asthma under control;
7 have my asthma reviewed at least once a year (more frequently if I have severe asthma) at a time convenient to me, or in the case of my children, every six months;
8 be referred to a respiratory specialist if my asthma is becoming unmanageable, and to be admitted to a specialist respiratory unit if I need to go to hospital;
9 have follow-up appointments made with my doctor and my specialist before I am discharged from hospital or leave A&E;
10 expect any people working in the NHS that I need to contact to be aware of the serious risks I face if my asthma symptoms are deteriorating (e.g. practice receptionists, ambulance personnel and NHS Direct staff).

If you substitute the words 'my child' for 'me' throughout the Charter you will get a clear picture of the standard of care your child should expect from health professionals.

Index

A&E departments 32–4
Action on Smoking and Health 60
acupressure 64
acupuncture 63–4, 72
additives 71
air ionizers 72
air pollution
  indoor 3–5, 7
  outdoor 2–3, 74
allergens 12, 40, 71
allergic illness/reaction 11, 13, 14, 56, 58
allergy testing 17–18
Allergy UK 23, 42
anaphylaxis 1, 14–15, 62
Anaphylaxis Campaign 15, 49, 62
animal dander 18, 19, 58
animals 1, 4, 8
anti-allergy bedding 19, 22, 42–3, 44
anti-allergy products 42–3
antibiotics 8, 29
anti-histamines 17, 26, 37, 46
anti-IgE monoclonal antibody 76
asthma
  attack, what to do in case of 27
  clinics 28, 30–1, 76
  and family life 40–6
  numbers of children with 1, 56
  prevention of 12, 17
  research into 73–7
  schools policy on 49–55
atopy 11, 58
Atrovent 37

babysitters 47
Becloforte 35
beclomethasone 35
Becotide 35, 65
breastfeeding 13, 15, 20, 65
breathlessness 1, 9, 10, 12, 13, 16, 17, 24, 36
Bricanyl 37
British Lung Foundation 2, 8, 73, 77

British Thoracic Society 3, 7, 11, 34, 57, 72
bronchiolitis 9, 10, 13, 19, 28, 56, 57
bronchodilators 9, 36–7, 57
budesonide 35
Buteyko 66–9, 72

career choices for asthmatics 61
cats 7–8, 17, 18
Cats Protection 24
chemical sensitivity 18
childcare 47
childminders 47–8
cigarette smoke 1, 4
climate 2
cold air 19, 25
cold virus 13, 19
complementary medicine 63–72
cookery lessons 48, 50
corticosteroids 35
cough 1, 9, 12, 16, 17, 24, 36
Cromogen 35
croup 10

damp dusting 23, 43
diagnosis, difficulties of 10, 28, 56, 57
diet 2, 5–6, 12, 20, 64–5, 70–3, 75

eczema 1, 12–15, 44
eformoterol 37
exercise 17, 19, 24–5, 50, 58, 71

family life 40
Flixotide 35
fluticasone 35, 39
food allergies 12, 19, 25, 44

genes 11
GP care 27–30

Hale Clinic 69
hay-fever 1, 12–14
HEPA filters 23, 41–2

herbal medicines 65–6, 70
heredity 11
holidays 43–6
homoeopathy 64, 70
house-dust mites 1–2, 4, 12, 18–19, 22–3, 40–1, 43, 44, 58
'Hygiene Hypothesis' 2, 7
hypnosis 72

Idling Immune System Theory 2, 6–7
immune system 12–14, 19
inhalers 37–9, 44, 46, 51–2, 65
   see also 'preventer' inhalers, and 'reliever' inhalers
Intal 35
ipratropium bromide 37

Leukotriene Receptor Antagonists 76
leukotrienes 66

mask 17, 30, 37–8

NAC holidays 44–6
NAC Scotland 32
National Asthma Campaign (NAC) 1, 23, 42, 43, 47, 52, 60, 63, 74, 76
National Childminding Association 48
National Institute of Medical Herbalists 65
nebulizer 17, 33, 37–8, 70
NHS Direct 27
nursery (school) 47–9

obesity 74
osteopathy 70
Oxis 37
ozone (levels) 3, 26

paracetamol 74
passive smoking 5, 19, 20–1, 57
peak flow 31
peanut allergy 12
pet hair 7
pets 12, 48, 50
Pill, the 8
playgroups 47–9
pollen 12, 18, 26, 50, 58
pregnancy 4–5, 8, 12, 57, 65, 73
premature babies 56, 73

Pre-School Learning Alliance 48
'preventer' inhalers 25, 29, 30, 35, 54, 57, 60, 63
Propolis 71
puberty 26, 56
Pulmicort 35
Pycnogenol 66

RAST test 41
reliever inhalers 25, 27, 29, 30, 35, 36, 50, 54, 57, 63
rhinitis 12
Royal Jelly 71

salbutamol 37
salmeterol 37, 39
school 47–55
science labs 50
Serevent 37
sleep problems 30, 32, 42
smoking 4, 13, 58, 73
sodium cromoglycate 35
spacers 17, 27, 30–1, 37–8
steroids 9, 13, 17, 29, 34, 36, 57, 65, 68–70, 76
   side-effects of 36
stress 19, 25, 67, 71
swimming 25

teenagers, asthma management for 59–62, 66, 76
terbutaline 9, 37
traffic fumes 3
'transient early wheezers' 56
triggers 1, 11, 16, 17–26

vaccination 8
vaccine 7, 74
Ventolin (inhaler) 17, 30, 37, 65, 68–9
viral-associated wheeze 10

weather 3, 26, 44
wheeze 1, 8, 9, 12, 13, 16, 17, 24, 29, 36, 65
world, asthma incidence 2

yoga 66–7, 72